Duty of Candour

When Things Go Wrong: Practising the Duty of Candour with Confidence

By

Daniel Meguille

E-Book: 979-8-9970285-0-3

Paperback: 979-8-9970285-1-0

Hardcover: 979-8-9970285-2-7

Table Of Contents

Preface

In the ever-changing, high-stakes world of healthcare, where decisions are made at the sharp edge of human vulnerability, the weight of responsibility carried by those who deliver care can be overwhelming. Every healthcare professional, whether a doctor, nurse, allied health practitioner, or manager, operates not only under the rigorous demands of knowledge and skill but also beneath an imperative to embody the highest standards of integrity and humanity. Amid the daily triumphs that define so much of clinical practice, there is the undeniable reality that sometimes, despite best intentions and utmost diligence, things will go wrong. These moments, painful and difficult, are the crucibles that test not only our competency but the moral fabric of healthcare itself.

It is within this profound and delicate space that the Duty of Candour takes centre stage. More than a policy mandate or a regulatory checklist, the Duty of Candour is a compass guiding us through the fog of uncertainty and distress when harm occurs. It calls on us to embrace transparency with humility and honesty, to engage in compassionate communication even when the easy path would be silence or obfuscation. This book invites you to explore this duty not as a burdensome obligation but as a vital act of respect for patients, families, and, indeed, us as professionals committed to healing.

As you open these pages, you will embark on a journey that blends legal and ethical frameworks with practical, actionable guidance. This is a book rooted in the realities of healthcare practice, informed by frontline experience, regulatory insight, and the voices of patients and families who have walked the painful road of adverse events. It is designed to equip you to respond with confidence and care when confronted with unsettling moments in which error or misfortune shadows the clinical encounter.

The themes woven throughout this work are as diverse as they are interconnected. Transparency and honesty lie at the heart, underscoring the essential truth that openness breeds trust, not only restoring relationships fractured by harm but also laying the groundwork for safer, more responsive care systems. Understanding the legal and ethical imperatives provides a sturdy foundation, clarifying why candour is not optional and helping to navigate the complex terrain where disclosure intersects with professional liability and organisational governance. Effective communication skills are explored in depth because candour is never merely about recounting facts; it is about empathetic dialogue that honours the dignity of those affected, validates their experiences, and paves the way for mutual understanding, even in adversity.

Learning and improvement are vital chapters in this story, reminding us that every incident of harm is a call to reflection and an opportunity to dissect what went wrong, why it happened, and how future occurrences might be prevented. It is not enough to say what went wrong; we must also commit to doing better. This commitment is inseparable from leadership and culture, which emerge as indispensable forces in transforming the abstract principles of candour into lived realities. The actions of leaders, the ethos they cultivate, and the support structures they build either nurture an environment where openness thrives or suffocate it beneath blame and fear.

Throughout the book, you will find real-world examples and thoughtfully crafted conversation scripts, templates, and policy tools designed to bring candour out of theory and into everyday clinical practice. These resources honour the complexity of human interaction and organizational dynamics, offering practical frameworks without robbing the conversation of its warmth and authenticity.

I hope that as you read, you will feel a growing sense of reassurance and empowerment. To practice the Duty of Candour is to acknowledge vulnerability, both ours as professionals and that of the people we serve. Yet within this vulnerability lies strength: the courage to speak truthfully, to listen openly, and to lead change. This is not simply about compliance or risk management; it is about embodying the spirit of patient-cantered care, of putting humanity at the core of healthcare.

This book is intended for every healthcare professional who faces those fragile moments when things unravel, those moments demanding honesty wrapped in kindness, integrity exercised with wisdom, and transparency balanced with sensitivity. It is for the managers and leaders whose vision and commitment create cultures were speaking up is welcomed, mistakes are seen as tools for learning, and trust is rebuilt steadily over time. It is for all who believe in a healthcare system that honours ethical responsibility as fiercely as clinical excellence.

In composing this work, I have been guided by the voices of many clinicians who have grappled with the aftermath of patient harm, the patients and families who have courageously shared their experiences, the regulators and legal experts who strive to align justice with fairness, and the leaders who champion a culture of openness even when it is far from easy. To them, I extend my deepest gratitude for their honesty, insight, and commitment.

As you turn these pages, may you feel less alone in the challenge of practicing candour. May you find in this book not only guidance and tools but also affirmation of the profound importance of your role in this noble and difficult enterprise. May it inspire you to transform moments of difficulty into opportunities for connection, learning, and hope so that care once wounded may heal with greater strength and grace. In the end, this is more than a duty: it is a promise to patients, to families, to us, and to the future of healthcare itself.

Welcome to "Duty of Candour: When Things Go Wrong Practising the Duty of Candour with Confidence." Let us begin this vital journey together.

Introduction:
Why Candour Matters

The Concept of Candour

At the heart of the healthcare journey lies a profound and often underestimated principle: candour. While the word itself may evoke images of simple honesty or straightforwardness, within the healthcare context, candour embodies something far more intricate and powerful. It is the deliberate commitment to openness and transparency when things go wrong, a pledge that demands not only truthfulness but also a depth of empathy, responsibility, and professional integrity. More than just a moral ideal, candour is a vital cornerstone on which the delicate, often fragile relationships between patients, families, and healthcare professionals are built and maintained. It is this unwavering dedication to truth that transforms clinical care from a cold exchange of services to a profoundly human interaction born of trust and respect.

Understanding candour requires us to first look beyond a simplistic binary of truth and deception. Candour is not merely about stating facts or admitting faults in a detached manner. It is an active process, a conscious choice to engage with patients and their families honestly about adverse events, mistakes, or harm, no matter how uncomfortable or challenging that may be. This process is not just about disclosures; it is about cultivating an environment where such openness is expected, cultivated, and supported. At its core, candour challenges the deeply rooted culture within many healthcare systems that has historically leaned toward silence, avoidance, or deflection when adverse events occur. It demands a shift that honours the humanity of all involved: the suffering patient, the conscientious clinician, and the often-bewildered family members by embracing transparency as an act of respect and care.

The relevance of candour reaches far beyond the immediate disclosure of an error or an unfortunate outcome. It strikes at the very foundation of trust, the sacred contract implicit in healthcare encounters. Patients enter relationships with clinicians not simply in exchange for treatment; they place their lives, dignity, and well-being in another's hands, hoping for competence, compassion, and truth. When things go wrong, confidence may falter, but it is candour that restores faith, reaffirming that the healthcare provider remains committed not only to healing but also to accountability and respect for the patient as a whole person. This restoration of trust is not merely an emotional balm; it is a critical factor in ongoing healing, better adherence to future care, and the overall patient experience.

Families, too, find solace in candour. They occupy a unique space of advocacy, support, and often helplessness when adverse events unfold. Their need to understand what happened, why it happened, and what will be done to prevent recurrence is deeply human. Transparency provides a bridge across the abyss of confusion and grief, turning opaque silence into a shared narrative of truth. When clinicians engage families with sincere openness, they foster collaborative partnerships that empower rather than alienate, easing the burden of uncertainty and making the path forward a joint endeavour grounded in honesty.

For clinicians and healthcare professionals, candour is both a professional obligation and a profound ethical commitment. It asks healthcare providers to confront the vulnerabilities of their practice and to embrace humility without fear of blame or retribution. This act of courage and authenticity serves as a counterweight to the high-pressure, risk-laden environments in which clinicians operate, a space where perfection is demanded but rarely achievable. By practicing candour, healthcare professionals not only maintain their integrity but also contribute to a culture in which learning and improvement thrive. This transformative approach reframes errors not as personal failings to be hidden but as opportunities to refine skills, improve systems, and enhance patient safety.

At the organizational level, instilling a culture of candour requires visionary leadership and steadfast policies that empower individuals to speak openly and without fear. It is a systemic commitment that extends beyond individual clinicians to encompass governance, training, and resource allocation. Healthcare organizations that prioritize candour create environments where staff feel supported in acknowledging mistakes, where transparency is embedded in clinical and administrative processes, and where patient safety is continuously pursued through shared learning. This cultural shift reduces the shame and stigma often associated with errors and promotes resilience not through silence, but through collective responsibility and openness.

Interestingly, candour also intersects deeply with legal and ethical frameworks that govern healthcare worldwide. While laws in various jurisdictions increasingly mandate truthful disclosure of adverse events, legal requirements alone do not capture the full spirit of candour. True candour encompasses the ethical dimensions of respect, dignity, and compassion, recognizing that legal compliance is only the floor, never the ceiling, of what patients and families deserve. The ethics of candour calls on clinicians not only to do what is legally obligatory but to act with kindness and humanity, transforming difficult conversations into meaningful exchanges of trust and reassurance.

Moreover, cherishing candour allows healthcare systems to harness the power of transparency as a driver for improvement. When adverse events and near misses are openly reported and discussed, organizations gain invaluable insights that fuel systemic learning. Errors cease to be hidden defects and instead become signposts highlighting areas that demand attention and innovation. This reflective practice not only reduces harm but also elevates the quality of care and respect patients receive. It creates a virtuous cycle in which openness nourishes safety, and safety reinforces trust, culminating in healthcare environments that are more resilient, compassionate, and patient-cantered.

The scope of candour, therefore, extends beyond the telling of the truth after an incident. It is woven into the entire fabric of healthcare practice, from everyday decision-making to crisis management, from individual bedside conduct to institutional policies. This book embarks on a journey to unpack this multifaceted concept, arming healthcare professionals and leaders not only with knowledge but with practical tools, compassionate communication strategies, and leadership insights necessary to embrace candour proactively. It aims to dismantle the fears and barriers that inhibit openness, replacing them with confidence and the courage to meet adversity with honesty and humanity.

Ultimately, embracing candour transforms difficult moments into opportunities for growth and healing. It propels healthcare professionals beyond defensive postures rooted in fear and into a realm of constructive engagement where trust is rebuilt, and patient safety is enhanced. This transformation benefits not only patients and families but clinicians themselves, fostering professional fulfilment rooted in integrity and sound ethics. As healthcare continues to evolve amidst increasing complexities and demands, the unwavering commitment to candour stands as an indispensable compass guiding decisions, shaping culture, and, above all, honouring the profound human connection at the heart of every healing encounter.

In stepping forward with candour, healthcare professionals affirm the promise that suffering shall not be met with silence, that every voice matters, and that truth is not a weapon but a pathway to healing. It is this promise that the pages ahead seek to illuminate, equipping readers to navigate the challenging yet rewarding journey of practising the Duty of Candour with confidence, compassion, and unwavering commitment.

Impact on Patients and Families

When healthcare goes awry, the ripple effects extend far beyond the immediate clinical environment. For patients and their families, encountering harm is not just a medical event; it often becomes a profound emotional upheaval. The experience of being injured or otherwise adversely affected by healthcare, whether through error, omission, or system failure, can shatter a person's sense of safety and well-being. In these moments of vulnerability, the way healthcare professionals respond is crucial. Openness, often crystallised in the practice of the Duty of Candour, serves as a lifeline for those affected, fostering healing, restoring dignity, and mending fractured trust. The impact of transparency, therefore, reaches deeply into the hearts and minds of patients and families, shaping not only their immediate reactions but also their long-term relationships with the healthcare system.

The experience of harm within healthcare is often traumatic, leaving patients and families with a complex blend of fear, confusion, anger, and grief. In many cases, the initial injury or mistake is only the beginning of a long emotional journey. Patients who have been harmed may find themselves grappling with questions that go unspoken and answers left unanswered. Families, standing beside their loved ones, often bear the double burden of concern for the patient's well-being and frustration over the lack of clear communication. In these fragile moments, transparency becomes far more than a procedural necessity; it is an expression of respect and humanity. When a healthcare professional embraces openness, acknowledging the event honestly and compassionately, patients and families feel seen and heard. This recognition validates their experience and lays the foundation for collaborative healing.

Openness in the face of harm fundamentally shifts the power dynamic that often exists in clinical settings. Historically, healthcare has sometimes been perceived as paternalistic, with providers as unquestioned authorities and patients relegated to passive recipients of care. When things go wrong, this imbalance can deepen, as patients may feel marginalised or dismissed. Yet, the Duty of Candour challenges this paradigm by promoting a relationship founded on honesty and shared understanding. By providing patients and their families with transparent information about what happened, why it happened, and what steps will follow, clinicians affirm their respect and partnership. This approach can alleviate feelings of helplessness and alienation, replacing them with empowerment and inclusion. Even when the news is difficult, patients and families often express gratitude for candour, perceiving it as a genuine effort to restore trust and accountability.

Trust, once fractured by adverse events, is a delicate and essential component of the healing process. When patients and families feel deceived or left in the dark, that breach can have long-lasting repercussions not only in their relationship with individual clinicians but in their confidence in the healthcare system. Conversely, honesty and transparency are powerful facilitators of trust rebuilding. Full disclosure allows patients to process the event's reality, ask questions, and receive answers that avoid ambiguity or evasion. This openness makes the difference between feeling betrayed and feeling cared for. Research has consistently shown that patients who receive timely, clear, and empathetic explanations after harm are more likely to maintain or even restore trust and are less inclined to pursue formal complaints or litigation. Beyond the individual case, a culture of transparency fosters an environment where safety and quality improvement flourish, further benefiting future patients.

The emotional impact of harm and the subsequent disclosure process also influence how patients and families cope with grief, loss, and uncertainty. Being harmed within a system designed to heal can engender feelings of profound shock and disillusionment. When the response to an adverse event includes openness, acceptance of responsibility, and empathetic communication, it acts as a therapeutic tool. Patients and families report that honest conversations help them make sense of their experiences, giving them a narrative that replaces confusion and fear with clarity and acceptance. It is within these conversations that clinicians could express sincere regret and convey humanity, offering apologies that are not just formulas but heartfelt acknowledgements of pain and harm. These interactions do not erase the incident but create meaningful space for emotional processing, validation, and, ultimately, hope.

Conversely, opacity or evasiveness in response to harm tends to magnify distress and mistrust. When patients and families perceive that information is being withheld or sugar-coated, uncertainty festers. This silence can compound the trauma, leading to prolonged feelings of anger, betrayal, and frustration. Family members may feel compelled to seek answers through complaints, legal action, or advocacy, which can strain relationships with healthcare providers and institutions. The ensuing adversarial atmosphere diverts attention from learning and improvement, damaging organisational reputations and morale. Importantly, the absence of candour undermines clinicians' professional identities, who may experience moral distress or guilt when forced to conceal mistakes. Thus, opacity not only harms patients and families but also reverberates throughout the healthcare system, highlighting why transparency must be embraced as a shared commitment.

The scope of impact on families is often underestimated, but no less significant. Families frequently act as advocates, caregivers, and emotional anchors during recovery from harm, navigating unfamiliar medical systems and complex information. Their need for transparent communication is especially acute because they carry the weight of supporting the patient while trying to comprehend what has happened. Open dialogue with healthcare teams not only helps families understand clinical details but also enables them to participate meaningfully in decisions about ongoing care and safety measures. This inclusivity fosters a sense of collaboration rather than confrontation. Moreover, when families feel respected and involved, they can become vital allies in system improvement, offering insights from their lived experience that might otherwise go unrecognized. In this way, transparency empowers families to move from helpless bystanders to active participants in safeguarding the quality of care.

The psychological burden borne by patients and families following an adverse event should never be underestimated. The trauma of harm is often compounded by the uncertainty of unanswered questions and the fear of recurrence. When healthcare providers fulfil the Duty of Candour with sensitivity and thoroughness, they not only fulfil an ethical and legal obligation but also contribute to psychological healing. Patients often recount how transparent conversations after adverse events helped them reconcile with what occurred, even when the outcomes were not favourable. The process of honest disclosure fosters an environment of trust, which can buffer against feelings of isolation, betrayal, and helplessness. Families, witnessing this openness, often find reassurance in the knowledge that the system acknowledges its fallibility, seeks accountability, and is committed to doing better. This dynamic can facilitate a gradual rebuilding of confidence in healthcare, which is crucial for continued engagement with necessary medical care.

Importantly, transparency grounds the healthcare encounter in fundamental ethical principles of respect and dignity. When harm occurs, acknowledging it openly respects patients and families as moral agents entitled to truth and information. This respect reinforces human dignity at a moment when individuals are most vulnerable, affirming their value beyond the role of a patient or statistic. It also serves as a collective acknowledgement within the healthcare community that errors and adverse events, while regrettable, are part of a larger human endeavour to heal and be accountable. In this way, the Duty of Candour acts as a moral compass, guiding clinicians towards integrity and compassion even amid difficult circumstances. This ethical stance strengthens the relational fabric of healthcare, nurturing empathy and understanding that ultimately support safer and more patient-centred care.

For many patients and families, transparency after harm also fulfils a deeply human need for closure. When the facts are laid bare, coupled with clear explanations and expressions of regret, families can begin to come to terms with the event and its consequences. This closure is critical not only for emotional healing but also for practical reasons. Understanding what occurred helps patients and families make informed decisions about ongoing treatment, rehabilitation, or legal matters. It can prevent unnecessary confusion or miscommunication that might otherwise prolong the trauma. Closure also breaks the cycle of blame and secrecy that undermines organisational learning. When information flows freely and respectfully, it enables healing conversations and sets the stage for meaningful improvements in care delivery.

The effects of openness extend beyond individual incidents into the broader culture of healthcare. When patients and families know that transparency is the norm, they approach interactions with greater confidence and reduced anxiety. This anticipatory trust encourages earlier and more frequent dialogue about risks, expectations, and outcomes, which in turn reduces the likelihood of surprises and misunderstandings. Patients feel safer voicing concerns or questions if they trust that clinicians will respond openly and honestly. Families become integral partners in care planning and safety monitoring, contributing to vigilant and responsive systems. Over time, openness reinforces a virtuous cycle wherein transparency leads to trust, trust fosters collaboration, and collaboration drives continuous improvement. This cultural transformation depends heavily on healthcare professionals committing to truthful communication, even when it is difficult.

At the heart of this commitment is the recognition that candour is not a one-off event but an ongoing relational process. For patients and families, being subjected to harm does not sever their fundamental need for connection and reassurance from those who care for them. Open disclosure practices ensure that dialogue continues beyond initial conversations, allowing concerns to be addressed as they arise and supporting sustained engagement in care. In this way, candour becomes a bridge across moments of uncertainty, preserving relationships that might otherwise falter. This continuity is especially important in complex cases requiring prolonged management, where trust and understanding can significantly influence outcomes and patient experience.

It is also vital to acknowledge the diversity of patient and family responses to disclosure. While many welcome transparency and information, others may experience distress or require additional support to process what has happened. Sensitivity to cultural backgrounds, health literacy levels, and individual emotional capacity is essential to tailor communication effectively. At times, patients or families may not initially want exhaustive details but still deserve honest acknowledgement of the event and assurance of ongoing attention. Healthcare professionals must navigate these nuances with empathy and flexibility, always prioritising dignity and respect. This adaptive approach helps ensure that openness strengthens rather than undermines the therapeutic alliance, meeting patients and families where they are.

Families' need for transparency also intersects with the broader implications of harm, including financial strain, changes in caregiving roles, and impacts on quality of life. Knowledge about what went wrong can guide families in accessing support services, legal advice, or compensation processes. It can also inform decisions about advocating for systemic changes or participating in broader patient safety initiatives. When healthcare providers openly share information and involve families in dialogue, they enable not only healing but empowerment. Patients and families become partners in a shared mission to enhance safety and prevent future harm, not just passive recipients of care but active agents of change. This collaborative spirit embodies the transformative potential of the Duty of Candour.

Ultimately, openness after harm affirms a fundamental truth of healthcare: that medicine, while powerful, is inherently human and fallible. Acknowledging imperfection does not diminish professionalism; indeed, it strengthens it by making space for learning, accountability, and compassion. For patients and families, bearing witness to this humility can be profoundly reassuring. It signals that clinicians and organizations are committed to doing right by those they serve, fostering a relationship of respect and trust even amid adversity. This transformative power of candour elevates it beyond policy or protocol; it becomes a moral imperative and a pathway to deeper healing for all involved.

To fail in candour is to risk compounding harm, damaging relationships, and obstructing progress. In contrast, ethical transparency offers patients and families a measure of control, understanding, and hope in their darkest moments. When healthcare professionals embrace the Duty of Candour, they not only comply with legal and professional standards but also commit to affirming the humanity of those they serve. This deep respect nourishes connection and trust, making candour a cornerstone of truly patient-centred care. As such, every healthcare professional must appreciate that the impact of transparency goes far beyond disclosure; it transforms suffering into stories of resilience, fear into faith, and harm into hope. In this profound way, openness is not merely a response to error but a powerful act of healing and reconciliation.

Benefits for Healthcare Professionals

Candour, often described as the foundation of truthful communication and openness in healthcare, brings profound and far-reaching benefits not only for patients and families but also, critically, for healthcare professionals themselves. Embracing the duty of candour is not solely an altruistic gesture aligned with ethical principles; it also serves as a protective and empowering framework for clinicians and healthcare teams. When professionals commit to transparency after adverse events or errors, they cultivate an environment in which trust is mutually reinforced, emotional burdens are alleviated, and professional growth is fostered. The often-overlooked personal and collective advantages of candour are pivotal in sustaining healthcare providers' morale, resilience, and capacity to learn from complex, high-pressure situations typical of modern clinical practice.

Foremost among the benefits for healthcare professionals is the enhancement of trust, not simply trust from patients and families, but the vital trust clinicians place in themselves and their peers. In the aftermath of a mistake or adverse event, clinicians frequently grapple with feelings of guilt, shame, and professional insecurity. These emotions, if left unaddressed, can lead to burnout, reduced job satisfaction, and emotional isolation, which can culminate in defensive practice or even attrition from the field. By openly acknowledging errors and engaging in honest dialogue with affected parties, professionals access an authentic pathway to resolution that helps restore their sense of integrity and self-respect. This restorative aspect of candour diminishes the corrosive impact of secrecy and fear, which too often exacerbate distress and impair performance. To embrace honesty is to affirm one's own commitment to high-quality care, reinforcing a personal and collective identity grounded in ethical responsibility rather than denial or evasion.

Furthermore, proficiency in practicing candour cultivates stronger interprofessional relationships and more cohesive healthcare teams. Transparency is contagious in the best sense; when one team member models open communication, it encourages others to follow suit, creating a ripple effect that promotes psychological safety within the clinical environment. Psychological safety, the shared belief that one can speak up and admit doubts or mistakes without retribution, is essential for effective teamwork and patient safety. Teams that embody candour are more likely to confront challenges collaboratively, report near misses, and support one another in learning from failures. This cultural shift away from blame towards collective responsibility fosters mutual respect, reduces conflict, and aligns the team's focus on continuous improvement instead of individual fault. Clinicians working within such supported networks tend to experience greater job satisfaction, decreased stress, and a renewed commitment to their roles.

The educational benefits of engaging openly in the duty of candour are substantial and contribute to lasting improvements in clinical practice. Each adverse event, when disclosed with candour and reviewed thoughtfully, becomes a powerful learning opportunity. Instead of incidents being hidden or minimized, they are examined in full transparency, enabling clinicians to identify root causes, systemic weaknesses, and preventive strategies. This improved insight informs evidence-based adjustments to protocols, training, and decision -making processes, ultimately enhancing patient safety and reducing the likelihood of recurrence. By participating in this transparent cycle of accountability and growth, healthcare professionals develop sharper critical-thinking skills and a better understanding of the complexities inherent in their work environment. The confidence gained from this rigorous yet compassionate approach to errors fosters not only improved judgment but also a more resilient professional identity that can adapt to and thrive in a demanding, dynamic field.

Beyond personal and team benefits, engaging proactively with the duty of candour strengthens professional integrity and public trust in healthcare. Healthcare workers occupy a privileged and often vulnerable position in society: they are entrusted with people's health, dignity, and lives. Upholding candour affirms this trust by demonstrating accountability and respect for patient autonomy and rights. This transparent stance protects healthcare professionals' reputations by preventing the erosion of trust caused by concealment or dishonesty, which can irreparably damage relationships and lead to prolonged legal repercussions or disciplinary actions. By opting for honesty, clinicians safeguard both their personal standing and their organizations' standing, reinforcing a culture in which ethical practice is the norm rather than the exception. The integrity preserved through candour also supports professionals in navigating medico-legal environments more effectively, making them less vulnerable to adverse consequences by demonstrating commitment to openness and responsibility immediately after incidents.

Moreover, adopting the duty of candour actively addresses the emotional and psychological well-being of healthcare providers, which is often underappreciated. The psychological distress generated by clinical adverse events, sometimes referred to as the "second victim" phenomenon, can cause acute stress reactions, anxiety, depression, and even post-traumatic stress disorder among clinicians. The path to recovery from such trauma is closely linked to how incidents are handled. When professionals feel compelled to hide or deny errors, they risk becoming trapped in cycles of guilt and isolation. By contrast, when they engage in honest conversations supported by organizational policies and leadership, they experience validation, compassion, and opportunity for closure. Honest disclosure allows professionals to share their burden with colleagues, patients, and families rather than carrying it silently, helping to mitigate feelings of shame. This shared vulnerability can strengthen emotional resilience and empower healthcare workers to continue delivering compassionate care despite the heavy demands of their roles.

The duty of candour further equips healthcare professionals with practical communication skills that are transferable beyond adverse event disclosures and improve overall patient interactions. Learning to navigate difficult conversations with empathy, clarity, and honesty enhances clinicians' ability to manage complex interpersonal dynamics, diffuse tension, and maintain therapeutic alliances. These skills foster stronger relationships with patients and families, not only during crises but throughout routine care. By practicing transparent dialogue, healthcare providers contribute to a culture of openness that demystifies healthcare processes for patients, improves adherence to treatment plans, and supports shared decision-making. This elevates the clinician's role and satisfaction by transforming care encounters into collaborative partnerships rather than hierarchical transactions marked by fear or suspicion.

Equally significant is how the duty of candour encourages healthcare professionals to engage in reflective practice, a cornerstone of professional development. Reflection after disclosure events prompts clinicians to evaluate not only the clinical aspects of care but also their own responses, communication styles, and emotional reactions. This systematic introspection nurtures continuous improvement and self-awareness, essential qualities for maintaining competence in an ever-evolving healthcare landscape. Those who embrace candour repeatedly develop a stronger capacity for humility and adaptability, critical traits for addressing future challenges with courage and clarity. The skills and attitudes cultivated through candour extend beyond individual improvement, fostering a collective ethos of transparency and lifelong learning within healthcare organisations.

In parallel, embracing candour has financial and organisational benefits that indirectly support healthcare professionals by improving workplace stability and resources. Transparent handling of incidents reduces the likelihood of costly litigation and regulatory sanctions, which can create significant stress and uncertainty for clinicians involved. Early open disclosure often facilitates resolution and reconciliation, minimising legal entanglements that otherwise divert precious time and energy from clinical work. Additionally, organisations committed to candour attract and retain staff who value ethical practice and professional support, helping reduce turnover and preserving team cohesion. Such environments offer healthcare professionals not only emotional and educational security but also a sustainable framework for delivering high-quality care without unmanageable pressures. The alignment of professional and organisational interests through candour creates a virtuous cycle that benefits patients and providers alike.

Importantly, the duty of candour also serves as a catalyst for leadership development among healthcare professionals. Being transparent after adverse events often places clinicians in positions where they must communicate difficult information, coordinate responses, and engage with multidisciplinary teams and organisational leaders. These experiences can accelerate the cultivation of leadership skills such as conflict resolution, emotional intelligence, and strategic thinking. Healthcare professionals who demonstrate competence and confidence in candour practices position themselves as trusted leaders and champions of patient safety initiatives within their organisations. This leadership role can be deeply fulfilling and offers an avenue to influence systemic change, amplifying the positive impact of transparency from individual incidents to institutional transformation.

Ultimately, the duty of candour is not merely about compliance or risk reduction; it is a transformative practice that enriches the professional lives of healthcare workers in multiple, interconnected ways. It restores their sense of purpose by reaffirming the ethical commitments underlying clinical care, builds resilience by enabling constructive responses to adversity, and empowers them through skill development and leadership opportunities. As professionals grow more comfortable with candour, they contribute to stronger, more compassionate healthcare cultures where mistakes become springboards for learning rather than sources of shame and division. This ongoing evolution supports not only safer patient outcomes but healthier, more supportive workplaces where clinicians and teams can thrive despite the inevitable challenges of their vocation.

In embracing the duty of candour with confidence and integrity, healthcare professionals assume an active role in shaping a future where transparency is ingrained, trust is swiftly rebuilt, and compassionate care remains at the heart of the patient journey. The personal and collective benefits of candid practice are thus both immediate and enduring, enhancing not only the care experience but also the very fabric of professional life. This book aims to guide you through that journey, equipping you with the knowledge, skills, and inspiration to meet the duty of candour as an essential component of your professional identity and a vital contributor to the healing process for patients, families, and indeed the healthcare professionals themselves.

Legal and Ethical Foundations

Statutory Requirements

Understanding the statutory requirements underpinning the Duty of Candour is essential for healthcare professionals who seek not only to comply with legal mandates but to embrace an ethical framework that supports transparency, accountability, and trust. The legal landscape governing the Duty of Candour varies across jurisdictions, yet converges on fundamental principles that prioritise patients' rights to honest communication following an adverse event and institutional obligations to ensure that such communication is timely, truthful, and compassionate. This convergence is deeply rooted in historic developments in medical law, evolving societal expectations about openness in healthcare, and a growing recognition that concealment or avoidance of candid dialogue can inflict further harm on patients and families, eroding trust in healthcare systems. Therefore, statutory requirements compel healthcare organisations and professionals to move beyond voluntary codes of conduct to legally binding duties, with clear consequences for non-compliance.

Within these statutory frameworks, candour is defined as an affirmative duty to disclose not only the occurrence of harm but also any associated errors, omissions, or shortcomings that contributed to the incident. This duty extends beyond mere factual reporting; it embodies an ethical commitment where honesty and empathy coexist with professional responsibility. Many jurisdictions have crystallised these principles into legislation that directly requires healthcare providers to inform patients and families candidly when things go wrong during care or treatment. The impetus for these laws often stems from high-profile cases in which a lack of openness exacerbated patient and public mistrust, as well as from landmark investigations revealing systemic failures to acknowledge and learn from harm. For instance, international inquiries into healthcare scandals have highlighted how secrecy and defensive practices compromise patient safety, thereby galvanising governments to enact legislation mandating transparent processes.

A foundational characteristic of statutory Duty of Candour obligations is that they are imposed on both individual healthcare professionals and healthcare organisations. While professional codes of conduct emphasise personal integrity, the statutes impose institutional accountability by mandating the establishment of policies, procedures, and training programs to foster an environment in which openness is the norm rather than the exception. Compliance is not optional; it is embedded within the standards of good practice that regulate licensing and accreditation. This multidimensional model ensures that candour is woven throughout all levels of care delivery, from the bedside clinician disclosing an adverse event to the organisational leadership fostering a culture that supports such disclosures. Thus, statutory provisions often require that healthcare providers promptly notify patients who have experienced harm, provide a substantive explanation of what went wrong, offer apologies where appropriate, and outline the steps being taken to investigate and prevent similar occurrences.

Ethical theories serve as a philosophical substratum reinforcing these legal commitments. The principle of veracity, a core medical ethic, insists on truth-telling as a moral obligation, grounded in respect for patient autonomy and dignity. The notion of beneficence further supports candour by promoting patients' best interests through honesty, enabling informed decision-making and psychological closure. Additionally, theories of justice underscore a patient's right to redress and fairness, which is compromised when information about harm is withheld. Modern bioethics thus paints the Duty of Candour not as a burdensome legal restriction but as an extension of fundamental values that elevate the patient-professional relationship beyond transactional care to one characterised by trust and mutual respect. Healthcare ethics bodies globally echo this sentiment, integrating statutory requirements with professional moral imperatives to create a seamless set of expectations that guide behaviour.

Examining the legal scaffolding reveals a patchwork of statutes, regulations, and codes, each with language but unified in intent. In jurisdictions such as the United Kingdom, the Health and Social Care Act 2008 (Regulated Activities) Regulations 2014 introduce a statutory Duty of Candour, requiring healthcare providers to disclose notifiable safety incidents to patients and caregivers in a timely, truthful, and comprehensible manner. This statute delineates specific thresholds of harm that trigger the duty and sets out procedural requirements, such as written notifications and documentation. Complementing this are professional codes from bodies such as the General Medical Council, which translate legal mandates into actionable principles for doctors, emphasising honesty in all circumstances and prescribing communication frameworks to minimise distress while honouring transparency. Similarly, in Australia, various states have incorporated Duty of Candour provisions within public health legislation and professional health practitioner acts, mandating disclosure and embedding compliance within licensure criteria. These legal instruments often co-exist with patient rights acts that affirm patients' entitlement to full and frank information about their care. Such multi-layered regulation reinforces the unwavering message that concealment of harm is incompatible with modern healthcare standards.

Diving deeper into case law further elucidates how courts have shaped and interpreted the scope of the Duty of Candour. Judicial decisions provide practical guidance on the extent of disclosure duties, exceptions, and the interplay with issues such as confidentiality and liability. Courts have underscored that the duty is not merely to disclose facts but to ensure that information is conveyed in a manner understandable to patients, accommodating their emotional and cognitive needs. Litigation histories reveal that failures to meet candour obligations can lead to findings of professional negligence or breach of statutory duty, often amplifying patient harm by complicating claims for redress. Conversely, cases demonstrate that transparent communication, timely apologies, and evidence of remedial action may mitigate legal repercussions and facilitate reconciliation. These judicial interpretations contribute to evolving legal standards, guiding healthcare professionals on practical boundaries and reinforcing that honesty itself is a legal safeguard, not just an ethical desideratum.

The interplay between Duty of Candour laws and other statutory frameworks also merits attention. For example, data protection and privacy laws such as the General Data Protection Regulation (GDPR) in Europe impose constraints on how patient information is shared but also provide exceptions that allow disclosures related to safety incidents when handled sensitively and lawfully. Similarly, whistleblowing statutes often complement candour requirements by protecting healthcare workers who report unsafe practices or breaches of the duty internally or to regulators. Understanding how these intersecting legal regimes function helps health professionals navigate complex situations with confidence, ensuring that compliance with the duty does not inadvertently contravene confidentiality or professional secrecy provisions. Moreover, statutory requirements frequently mandate that healthcare providers cooperate with regulatory bodies during investigations, balancing candour with respect for procedural justice and legal rights.

One of the most pivotal parts of the statutory Duty of Candour is the mandated incorporation of apology as a legal element. Apologies serve multiple functions: they acknowledge harm, express regret, and can begin healing fractured relationships. Recognising this, many statutes clarify that expressions of regret or apologies made in good faith are not admissible as evidence of admission of liability in subsequent legal proceedings, thereby encouraging openness without increasing legal risk. This delicate balance encourages healthcare providers to meet ethical and statutory expectations without fear that candid words will be weaponised in litigation against them. In many cases, these legislative provisions have catalysed a cultural shift where apology is no longer viewed solely as an admission of fault but as a necessary component of patient-centred care and candour.

Crucially, statutory requirements often extend beyond the immediate communicative exchange to encompass systemic obligations. These include the duty to investigate incidents thoroughly, report findings to relevant oversight agencies, and implement measures to prevent recurrence. Health organisations are required to maintain records demonstrating compliance with the duty, facilitating audits and enforcement actions. This institutional angle reflects society's expectation that candour is not a passive reaction but part of an active quality assurance and risk management framework. Ensuring that statutory obligations are met entails robust training, support for healthcare workers to manage emotionally charged disclosures, and leadership commitment to transparency. Failure to embed these practices may render compliance superficial and ultimately ineffectual, risking sanctions ranging from fines to reputational damage and, in severe cases, criminal prosecution.

Despite the clarity of statutory mandates, practical challenges arise when applying these laws in diverse clinical settings. For example, determining which incidents meet the disclosure threshold can be complex, especially in high-acuity environments where adverse outcomes may be multifactorial. Moreover, cultural nuances concerning truth-telling, especially in multicultural societies, can affect how candour is perceived and enacted. Statutory frameworks thus sometimes incorporate flexibility to respect individual circumstances and informed patient preferences, while still emphasising the non-negotiable principle of honesty. Equipping healthcare professionals with comprehensive legal and ethical education helps them interpret and implement the duty with sensitivity and consistency, reducing the risk of inadvertent breaches or defensive behaviours that impede openness.

Healthcare regulators play a pivotal role in ensuring that statutory Duty of Candour requirements are not viewed as abstract legalities but as living commitments embedded in everyday practice. Through standards enforcement, audits, and feedback mechanisms, regulatory bodies monitor organisational compliance, facilitate learning from incidents, and, where necessary, impose sanctions. These agencies often provide guidance documents, toolkits, and training resources that translate statutory language into operational protocols, thus bridging the gap between legal theory and practice. Collaboration between healthcare organisations, regulators, and professional bodies fosters a shared understanding of statutory duties, aligned incentives for transparent behaviour, and joint efforts to embed candour in healthcare cultures worldwide.

In sum, the statutory requirements surrounding the Duty of Candour constitute a complex but coherent framework that legally mandates healthcare transparency following adverse events. This framework is woven together by both legislative texts and professional codes, informed by ethical theory and judicial interpretation, and situated within a broader ecosystem of related laws and regulatory oversight. For clinicians and healthcare managers alike, understanding these obligations is paramount to fulfilling their professional roles with integrity and compassion. The laws not only compel disclosure to safeguard patient rights and public trust but also encourage an organisational ethos where openness is integral to clinical excellence and patient safety. Far from being merely a set of rules, the statutory Duty of Candour represents a transformative commitment to honesty in healthcare, one that, when embraced wholeheartedly, enhances healing, learning, and justice for all involved.

Ethical Principles

Honesty stands as the bedrock of ethical conduct in healthcare, encompassing more than a mere expectation or procedural formality; it serves as the moral compass guiding interactions among clinicians, patients, and their families during the most vulnerable and challenging moments. In embracing honesty, healthcare professionals commit to transparency that nurtures trust, which is essential for the therapeutic alliance and for safeguarding the dignity and autonomy of those in their care. This commitment is not simply a passive avoidance of deception; rather, it demands an active and deliberate willingness to disclose information fully and candidly, even when such disclosure risks discomfort, legal exposure, or personal distress. It manifests as openness about errors, adverse outcomes, and uncertainties, reflecting an ethical imperative grounded in respect for the patient's right to know and participate meaningfully in decisions about their health and wellbeing. Honesty in this context is intertwined with the principle of truth-telling, an unwavering stance that fosters integrity and personal accountability from healthcare professionals and lays the groundwork for restoring confidence after the inevitable lapses that occur in complex medical systems.

Accountability in healthcare, as an ethical pillar, extends this dimension of honesty into the realm of responsibility. It calls upon clinicians and healthcare organisations not only to acknowledge mistakes but to own them unequivocally, refraining from defensiveness or denial. This ethical notion is more than an admission of fault; it embodies an obligation to act in ways that promote learning, correction, and the prevention of future harm, binding at both the individual and systemic levels of practice. Accountability requires professionals to reflect critically on their actions, employing humility to recognise fallibility while maintaining a steadfast commitment to improvement. Embedded within this principle is an acknowledgement that healthcare is an inherently social endeavour, an exchange where the consequences of actions ripple beyond the individual clinician to affect patients, families, and communities. Thus, accountability also demands transparency to regulatory bodies and the public, thereby entrenching trust not only in personal conduct but also in the healthcare system's capacity for self-regulation, correction, and growth.

Respect serves as a transcendent ethical principle that guides how honesty and accountability are enacted in healthcare encounters. It is a multifaceted concept encompassing recognition of the inherent worth and dignity of patients as autonomous agents with unique values, preferences, and experiences. Respect shapes how candid conversations are conducted, emphasising empathy, cultural sensitivity, and the delicate stewardship of information. Through respectful communication, healthcare professionals honour patients' agency by providing truthful information in a manner that is comprehensible, compassionate, and responsive to their needs and emotions. Respect also entails acknowledging the moral distress that both patients and clinicians may experience in the wake of adverse incidents, cultivating space for expression, validation, and dialogue. This mutual respect serves as a crucial counterbalance to the potential anxieties of disclosure, fostering an environment where honesty can flourish without fear of judgment or retribution, thereby reinforcing relational trust and shared commitment to healing.

The ethical foundation of the Duty of Candour is deeply rooted in classical moral philosophies while evolving to meet the complex realities of modern healthcare. The principle of beneficence, which obliges clinicians to act in patients' best interests, inevitably entails an obligation to be truthful, as patients require accurate information to make decisions that promote their welfare. Simultaneously, non-maleficence, the duty to do no harm, imposes a mandate to promptly reveal adverse events to mitigate further injury, acknowledge suffering, and enable appropriate remedial actions. Honesty and transparency thus serve as practical extensions of these foundational precepts, transforming abstract moral duties into concrete clinical responsibilities. Kantian ethics, with its emphasis on treating persons as ends in themselves rather than as means, reinforces the moral necessity of truthful disclosure as an expression of respect for patient autonomy and dignity. It challenges healthcare professionals to act according to maxims that could be universally willed, including the commitment to candour, even when such honesty may carry personal or institutional risk.

Conversely, utilitarian ethics, centred on the greatest good for the greatest number, points toward honesty as a mechanism to enhance overall patient safety through systemic learning and prevention of recurrent harm. Transparent disclosure of incidents fosters an environment of openness that supports robust quality improvement initiatives, reduces errors, and promotes equitable care. The ethical tension between these theories is vivid when balancing individual patient interests with broader organisational imperatives; nonetheless, transparency consistently emerges as a shared value that prioritises trust and the minimisation of suffering. Virtue ethics further enriches this discourse by emphasising moral character traits such as courage, integrity, and humility, which enable healthcare professionals to confront difficult truths and engage in meaningful reflection. Courage underpins the strength required to disclose errors honestly, especially within hierarchical or blame-oriented contexts, while humility permits acceptance of fallibility, empowering professionals to embrace learning opportunities rather than conceal mistakes.

In addition to these ethical theories, contemporary frameworks emphasise relational ethics, which foregrounds the significance of relationships and context in ethical decision-making. The Duty of Candour embodies relational ethics through its insistence on openness and empathy, recognising that ethical disclosure is not a detached procedural formality but a deeply interpersonal act. This approach accounts for the complexity of individual circumstances, varying patient expectations, and cultural diversities that shape how candour is received and interpreted. It situates honesty within a dynamic exchange of trust, vulnerability, and moral responsiveness, requiring healthcare professionals to attend sensitively to patients' and families' narratives, emotions, and information needs. Consequently, ethical candour transcends rigid mandates and becomes an embodied practice that balances fidelity to professional duties with compassion and contextually attuned communication.

The statutory underpinnings of the Duty of Candour across various jurisdictions crystallise these ethical principles into legal obligations, intertwining professional standards with public accountability. For instance, in England, the Health and Social Care Act 2008 (Regulated Activities) Regulations 2014 institutionalise the Duty of Candour, mandating healthcare providers to notify patients of 'notifiable safety incidents' promptly and to provide reasonable support during and after disclosure. This statute codifies honesty, accountability, and respect into actionable requirements, reinforcing the ethical imperative with legal force. Similarly, in Scotland, the Healthcare Improvement Scotland (Duty of Candour) Regulations 2018 delineate parallel duties, emphasising timely, truthful communication and fostering a culture of openness. In these frameworks, failure to comply can carry significant reputational and regulatory consequences, underscoring the seriousness with which transparency is regarded. Such legal provisions serve to protect patients' rights, enhance safety, and promote system-wide learning, thus operationalising the ethical call for candour into enforceable standards

Professional codes of conduct further enshrine these ethical foundations, providing detailed guidance on how honesty and accountability should be practised in clinical settings. The General Medical Council (GMC), for example, outlines in its Good Medical Practice guidance that doctors must be honest and open, especially when things go wrong, including offering an apology and explaining the facts as far as they are known. The Nursing and Midwifery Council (NMC) similarly codifies expectations for nurses to act with integrity and promote a culture of openness and honesty. These codes articulate not only aspirational virtues but also concrete behaviours and responsibilities, articulating that ethical conduct demands both principled commitment and practical application. They bind individual practitioners to uphold transparency as a professional norm, serving both as ethical compasses and benchmarks for accountability within disciplinary frameworks. Importantly, these codes recognise the emotional and ethical challenges inherent in practising candour, encouraging ongoing education, peer support, and reflective practice as means to strengthen moral resilience and competence.

Judicial rulings and case law offer additional insight into how these ethical principles are interpreted and enforced, especially in contentious or complex scenarios. Courts have increasingly emphasised the patient's right to be informed about healthcare incidents, sometimes ruling that failure to disclose material information breaches the duty of care and constitutes negligence. Landmark cases have reinforced that honest communication and apology do not equate to admissions of legal liability but rather align with ethical and legal duties, encouraging openness without exacerbating adversarial dynamics. Such jurisprudence has developed alongside statutory reforms, creating a jurisprudential landscape that strengthens the protection of patients' rights and incentivises candour. The judiciary also recognises the delicate balance between transparency and safeguarding the interests of healthcare professionals and institutions, navigating these tensions with sensitivity to promote trust and systemic improvement rather than punitive measures. This evolving body of law thus reflects societal values that prize honesty, accountability, and respect, embedding these ethical principles more firmly in healthcare governance.

Understanding the interplay between these ethical principles and their regulatory embodiments equips healthcare professionals with the contextual clarity needed to fulfil their Duty of Candour confidently and competently. Awareness of the moral weight of honesty, accountability, and respect transcends compliance, transforming duty from a distant mandate into a lived commitment that enhances professional identity and patient-centred care. Integrating these principles into everyday practice fosters an ethical climate that not only responds to incidents transparently but proactively cultivates trust, reduces blame, and promotes continuous learning. It empowers healthcare professionals to navigate the emotional complexities of disclosure with compassion, moral courage, and reflective insight. Moreover, by embracing these ethical foundations, clinicians and leaders contribute to reshaping organisational cultures, dismantling fear and secrecy, and championing a healthcare environment where openness and humanity prevail.

In essence, the ethical principles of honesty, accountability, and respect form the triadic axis upon which the Duty of Candour is anchored. They compel healthcare professionals to undertake the vulnerable but vital journey toward truthfulness, assuming responsibility not merely as technical experts but as moral agents entrusted with the care and dignity of patients. This ethical framework challenges systems to transcend procedural responses and cultivate genuine relationships grounded in transparency and trust. By embodying these principles, healthcare professionals become architects of a safer, more compassionate, and just healthcare environment, one where candour is neither feared nor avoided but embraced as the cornerstone of ethical practice and healing.

Professional Codes and Standards

Within the realm of healthcare, the imperative to embody candour, the decisive commitment to openness, honesty, and transparency when adverse events occur, is not merely an aspirational ideal but a firmly embedded professional obligation codified through an array of codes, standards, and guiding principles promulgated by medical and nursing bodies worldwide. These professional frameworks provide healthcare practitioners with an essential compass, directing behaviour in moments fraught with ethical complexity and emotional turbulence. They articulate expectations for conduct that transcend regulatory mandates, imbuing the practice of candour with moral force derived from foundational principles such as beneficence, non-maleficence, autonomy, and justice. A deep understanding of these professional codes is paramount, for they distil decades of ethical reflection, learned experience, and legal requirements into practical guidance tailored for those on the frontlines of care.

Medical bodies, such as the General Medical Council (GMC) in the United Kingdom, the American Medical Association (AMA) in the United States, the Canadian Medical Association (CMA), and similar authorities globally, emphasise the centrality of honesty and transparency in their codes of ethics and guidelines on professional conduct. The GMC's "Good Medical Practice" explicitly mandates that doctors be open and honest with patients when things go wrong and apologise where appropriate, setting a clear expectation that candour is integral to maintaining trust and safeguarding patient welfare. This overt prescription reinforces that disclosure is not optional or circumstantial but a core facet of professional responsibility. The AMA's Code of Medical Ethics echoes these sentiments, articulating that physicians should disclose errors to patients and families in a timely, empathetic manner, while balancing the need to maintain professionalism and manage legal considerations prudently. The emphasis across these documents consistently underscores that truthfulness in the face of adverse outcomes is a hallmark of medical professionalism and an ethical non-negotiable.

Nursing bodies similarly enshrine candour within their professional codes, recognising the distinct role nurses play as patient advocates and trusted caregivers who frequently serve as intermediaries between the healthcare system and the individual receiving care. The International Council of Nurses (ICN) Code of Ethics stresses the nurse's responsibilities to prioritise patient safety and well-being, which intrinsically includes transparent communication about risks, mistakes, and the measures being taken to address harm. National nursing associations, such as the Royal College of Nursing (RCN) in the UK and the American Nurses Association (ANA) in the US, further elaborate on these principles by providing detailed protocols that guide responses to adverse events. These frameworks underscore the importance of honesty, not only as a matter of ethics but as an essential ingredient in fostering therapeutic relationships grounded in respect and dignity. Nurses are also encouraged to document disclosures thoroughly and to engage with interdisciplinary teams to ensure systemic learning from errors, thereby linking individual candour to broader organisational accountability.

What resonates powerfully across these bodies is the framing of candour not merely as an isolated communication act but as an ethical continuum encompassing transparency before, during, and after incidents, as well as ongoing engagement with patients and families. It is a relational process that requires practitioners to navigate the delicate balance between openness and professional discretion, to acknowledge harm without evading responsibility, and to sustain compassion even in the shadow of failure or unforeseen outcomes. Such a nuanced ethical stance is buttressed by a range of ethical theories that have shaped modern healthcare professions. Principles, with their pillars of autonomy, beneficence, non-maleficence, and justice, validate the imperative of candour, as respect for patient autonomy requires full disclosure of the information matrices that affect decision-making. From a virtue ethics perspective, candour is an expression of integrity, courage, and humility, the traits that define a trustworthy practitioner who places patient welfare above concerns of reputation or litigation.

Deontological ethics emphasises duties and rules, reinforcing the view that honesty constitutes a binding professional and moral obligation regardless of the consequences. Conversely, utilitarianism supports candour on pragmatic grounds, advocating transparency to enhance patient safety, improve systems, and prevent future harm, thereby maximising overall good. The amalgamation of these ethical underpinnings buttresses the position that the duty of candour is a multidimensional construct, deeply embedded in the moral fabric of healthcare professions and reflective of a commitment not just to truth-telling, but to repairing trust and promoting justice.

In tandem with ethical codes, legal frameworks in various jurisdictions have increasingly codified the duty of candour, intertwining professional standards with statutory mandates. For instance, the UK's Health and Social Care Act 2008 and subsequent regulations impose statutory obligations for healthcare providers to notify patients and their families candidly about incidents causing harm, supported by oversight from regulatory bodies such as the Care Quality Commission (CQC). These legislative measures reflect a societal recognition that healthcare institutions bear collective accountability and that professional honesty is essential to the system's integrity and patient protection. Moreover, case law in many countries has gradually affirmed that failure to provide full and truthful information can constitute negligence or a breach of statutory duties, thereby reinforcing professional codes by attaching legal consequences to violations of candour obligations.

International variations in legal contexts require practitioners to be attuned not only to broad ethical principles but also to the specifics of national regulations and institutional policies. Nonetheless, the core message from medical and nursing professional bodies remains remarkably consistent: candour is not an ancillary or discretionary element of practice, but a fundamental duty entrenched in the professional identity of healthcare workers. Such codes frequently provide clear directives on practical aspects of disclosure, such as the need for timely communication, documenting conversations, providing support to patients and staff, and collaborating with regulatory authorities. They also acknowledge challenges, including fear of litigation, cultural resistance within organisations, and the emotional burden on professionals, and advise strategies to address them without compromising the imperative of honesty.

A further dimension emphasised in these codes concerns the maintenance of professional boundaries and emotional resilience when practising candour. Healthcare providers are encouraged to approach disclosures with empathy and sensitivity while safeguarding their own well-being through reflective practice, supervision, and institutional support systems. This recognition of the emotional complexity inherent in transparent communication highlights the progressive humanisation of professional mandates, portraying candour as an act of moral courage that requires both personal strength and ethical clarity.

Importantly, these professional codes and standards serve a dual function: they instruct practitioners on how to uphold the duty of candour in accordance with ethical and practical frameworks, and they also protect patients by embedding transparency as a safeguard against concealment or denial of harm. This reciprocal relationship fosters mutual trust, critical to therapeutic relationships and systemic learning. It signals an evolving healthcare culture, one that increasingly values openness, accountability, and continuous improvement as cornerstones of patient safety and quality care.

Healthcare professionals equipped with a robust understanding of these codes will find themselves better prepared not only to comply with technical requirements but also to internalise candour as an ethical commitment that enriches their practice. By familiarising themselves with the guidance from medical and nursing regulatory bodies, practitioners can navigate the complexities of adverse event disclosure with confidence, clarity, and compassion, transforming difficult moments into meaningful opportunities for healing and progress. The necessity of continuous engagement with professional updates, reflective learning, and organisational support further ensures that the duty of candour remains a living principle, dynamically responsive to evolving challenges and contexts. Ultimately, these layers of professional guidance and ethical reflection coalesce to form a sturdy foundation on which healthcare professionals can stand firm, knowing that openness is not merely mandated but embodies the very essence of responsible, patient-centred care.

Immediate Response: First Steps After an Incident

Securing Patient Safety

In the vital moments following an adverse event in healthcare, the paramount concern must invariably be securing patient safety. This responsibility is immediate and unambiguous: it transcends all other considerations and sets the foundation upon which every subsequent action is built. When things go wrong, the instinct to safeguard the patient, to stabilise their condition, and to prevent further harm must guide all professionals regardless of the complexity of the incident or the pressures of time. Securing patient safety is not merely a procedural task; it is a solemn duty rooted in the very ethics of caregiving and the trust placed in healthcare providers. The initial moments after an incident are often chaotic, fraught with emotional turmoil and confusion, yet it is within this space that clarity of purpose and rapid, decisive action can change the trajectory from further deterioration to controlled resolution.

The process begins with rapid assessment and immediate intervention, a phase where the clinical team must focus solely on the patient's current condition. This involves not only recognising signs of distress or deterioration but also mobilising any available resources to stabilise vital functions. The clinician must perform a thorough, swift examination to identify any life-threatening complications, recognising that time is often unforgiving. Whether the harm is physical, such as a medication error causing an allergic reaction, or procedural, such as a postoperative bleed, the priority is to arrest any trajectory that could worsen the patient's condition. This do-or-die focus on patient stabilisation demands calm leadership and a clear chain of command within the healthcare team, where roles are immediately understood and executed without hesitation. During this time, distractions like documentation or communication with family members, however important, must yield to the primacy of clinical care.

Equally important in securing patient safety is the early identification and mitigation of risks that could compound harm. This includes identifying and mitigating environmental hazards, ensuring the patient's surroundings are safe and secure to prevent falls or other accidents. It extends to reviewing the medication administration process, verifying dosages, and halting any treatments that could contribute to adverse reactions. Engaging pharmacy staff or specialists promptly can provide crucial insight to avert cascading complications. Similarly, teamwork at this stage is essential. Nurses, doctors, allied health staff, and, where available, rapid response teams must synchronise their efforts to not only treat but also continuously monitor the patient. This coordinated vigilance ensures that new risks do not emerge unnoticed in the immediate aftermath of the event.

While attention to the patient's physical condition dominates the initial response, healthcare staff must also address the psychological impact on the patient and their family. Securing patient safety expands beyond the corporeal to encompass emotional safety, which is critical in maintaining trust and confidence. A patient who feels cared for holistically will be more likely to collaborate with care providers and less prone to distress that could complicate recovery. This aspect requires professionals to communicate briefly, calmly, and honestly about what is being done, reassuring the patient with presence and empathy, even if full disclosure is reserved for a later, more considered conversation. Simple acts of kindness, such as sitting at the bedside, offering fluids, or providing a comforting touch where appropriate, can create a profound sense of security in a moment rife with vulnerability.

Once immediate clinical needs are addressed, the focus on securing patient safety shifts to ensuring ongoing monitoring and documentation. This is not a passive process but an active vigilance in which changes in the patient's condition must be detected early and escalated without delay. Healthcare professionals must not only rely on their senses and clinical intuition but also deploy appropriate monitoring technologies and protocols to flag deterioration. Meticulous recording of vital signs, responses to interventions, and any unusual symptoms is essential, as this information forms the cornerstone for both ongoing clinical management and transparent communication about the incident. Documenting actions taken to safeguard the patient also establishes a clear timeline and forensic trail that will support subsequent investigations and quality improvement efforts.

The initial securing of safety also entails promptly notifying relevant stakeholders within the healthcare setting. Early reporting to supervisors, risk managers, and clinical governance leads activates systems designed to support both the patient and the professionals involved. This internal alert triggers cascade mechanisms for further review, mobilising resources such as incident reporting teams, patient safety officers, and, where necessary, specialist consultants. Such notification is not about assigning blame but about rallying a collective response to stabilise the situation and prevent recurrence. The culture of transparency that underpins the Duty of Candour must be mirrored in these internal communications, where honesty and openness encourage learning over defensiveness. When team members feel supported rather than judged, they are more likely to contribute fully to mitigation efforts.

Alongside internal notifications, securing patient safety also demands readiness to engage external parties when required. In certain contexts, this might mean rapid involvement of emergency services or transfer to higher-acuity care facilities. Alternatively, regulators or patient representatives may need prompt communication, not to complicate the situation but to ensure that support systems external to the immediate care team are activated early. The choice of whom to notify and when should be guided by clearly established protocols grounded in patient welfare, legal requirements, and ethical obligations. Delays or failures in these steps compromise not only the safety of the individual patient but also the integrity of the healthcare organisation, eroding public trust and exposing professionals to avoidable liability.

In securing patient safety, the dynamics of teamwork and leadership are critically amplified. Effective response relies heavily on a culture in which staff feel empowered to act decisively and raise concerns without fear. Leadership presence during these moments can anchor the team, provide clarity of purpose and reinforce the importance of both clinical and communicative measures. Leaders act as both coordinators and moral compasses, reminding everyone involved that avoiding further harm is the collective priority and that transparency will follow naturally once the patient is secure. They must also recognise and address the emotional toll that acute incidents take on staff, as unresolved stress can impair judgment and reduce the quality of care delivered. Supportive leadership, thus, is a linchpin in transforming an adverse event from a crisis into an opportunity for responsible action and eventual recovery.

Another critical consideration in securing patient safety is the potential for systemic issues that may have contributed to the incident. While immediate attention focuses naturally on the patient and the event's direct effects, astute professionals begin to observe for signs of broader patterns, whether in protocols, environment, equipment, or human factors that could pose ongoing dangers. Identifying these early clues during initial response can inform the urgency and scope of subsequent investigations and corrective actions. Essentially, safeguarding the patient in the moment also means protecting future patients by starting to unravel preventable risks embedded in the system. This approach requires keen observational skills and a willingness to report even seemingly minor irregularities as part of the comprehensive safety strategy.

The act of securing patient safety is closely intertwined with the need to gather accurate, objective information about what has occurred. While this step can seem challenging, especially when emotions run high and the clinical environment is saturated with urgency, it is essential to approach the collection of facts methodically and sensitively. Immediate actions like stabilising the patient cannot be compromised, but as soon as the situation permits, careful and unbiased documentation of the timeline, personnel involved, and clinical notes takes place. This foundation of factual clarity supports not only medical continuity but also the transparency that patients and families expect in the aftercare dialogue. It prevents assumptions and miscommunications from taking root, which can otherwise undermine trust and complicate resolution. Practitioners must balance the urgency of information gathering with the compassion required in delicate circumstances, ensuring accuracy does not come at the cost of empathy.

Moreover, securing patient safety after an adverse event holds a powerful message to patients and families: that the healthcare team is wholly committed to their well-being, even when complications arise. This commitment must be evident in every action from the moment the event occurs. Patients who witness the swift and thorough mobilisation of care are more likely to feel valued and protected, which can mitigate some of the distress and fear that accompany harmful incidents. Conversely, if safety feels compromised or relegated to secondary status, distrust and dissatisfaction invariably follow, spilling over into litigation or a loss of reputation. Thus, the ethical imperative to secure patient safety is also foundational to the relational contract of healthcare, where openness and protection reinforce each other in a cycle that promotes healing beyond physical recovery.

Finally, the priority on securing patient safety within the duty of candour framework should never be seen as an isolated task performed solely by frontline caregivers. It is an organisational responsibility, supported by clear policies, training, and resources that enable swift and effective action. Healthcare institutions must cultivate environments where every team member understands their role in immediate response, where drills and education prepare staff for critical moments, and where safety equipment and protocols are accessible and up to date. This broad approach ensures that securing safety is not reliant on chance or individual heroism but is embedded in the fabric of care delivery. By investing in these systemic supports, organisations create the conditions for confident, compassionate, and transparent responses when things go wrong, reducing harm and strengthening trust for all who depend on healthcare services.

Fact Gathering and Incident Assessment

In the moments following an adverse event, healthcare professionals are thrust into a critical phase where the immediacy of action converges with the necessity for precision. The process of fact gathering and incident assessment is pivotal, not merely as a bureaucratic step but as the foundation for all subsequent responses, clinical, legal, ethical, and communicative. It is an exercise demanding agility, sensitivity, and unwavering commitment to accuracy. When harm has occurred or is suspected, rapidly collecting accurate information is both a moral imperative and a practical necessity, shaping the trajectory of patient safety, trust restoration, and organisational integrity. Yet, it is not simply the speed that counts; the quality and completeness of the information must be safeguarded amidst the urgency.

From the first acknowledgement of an incident, the healthcare professional's focus must be crystal clear, prioritising the patient's immediate safety and wellbeing. This includes stabilising the patient, if necessary, and ensuring that no further harm occurs while the factual landscape is mapped diligently. This dual focus, caring for the patient's physical condition while concurrently beginning systematic fact-finding, presents a challenge that underlines the complexity of the clinician's role. The initial response sets the tone for all that follows. How open, how transparent, and how empathetic the entire process will be is often determined by the approach taken in these formative moments.

Effective fact gathering begins with observing and recording the immediate circumstances surrounding the incident without delay. The environment itself is a critical source of insight; lighting, equipment placement, patient positioning, and the presence or absence of emergency interventions all contribute essential context. Healthcare professionals are advised to note these details as soon as possible, while they remain fresh in memory, taking care to preserve the scene where feasible, mindful of both patient comfort and clinical urgency. This early capture helps prevent the loss or distortion of facts that can occur under pressure or over time.

An accurate, contemporaneous account from the involved healthcare staff is invaluable. Gathering narratives from those directly participating or witnessing the event must be handled with tact and impartiality. The objective is not to assign blame instantly, but to reconstruct what occurred as faithfully as possible. This can be complicated by the natural human inclination toward self-preservation or defensiveness, as well as by differing perceptions of the event. Encouraging an open, non-judgmental atmosphere where individuals feel supported to share their observations fosters honesty and reduces the risk of crucial information being withheld. Those involved must understand that fact gathering serves the patient's interests foremost and the collective goal of improving safety rather than penalising errors.

Alongside human accounts, an examination of clinical documentation and electronic health records is critical. Precise review of medication charts, nursing notes, care plans, and monitoring data may reveal discrepancies, omissions, or trends that illuminate the incident. While documentation is often extensive and complex, it can reveal subtle clues: timing of medication administration, changes in vital signs, or delays in care escalations. Extracting and interpreting this data requires both clinical acumen and procedural knowledge, underscoring the importance of early multidisciplinary involvement. For example, pharmacists, nursing supervisors, and clinical governance personnel can enrich the fact-finding process by lending their expertise and an additional layer of oversight.

It is equally important to identify and review any material or equipment implicated in the incident. Whether a malfunctioning device, an expired medication, or a compromised supply item, physical evidence can sometimes provide undeniable answers or highlight system weaknesses that contributed to the event. Ensuring such items are preserved and assessed promptly can prevent contamination or loss and is often critical for both internal investigations and potential regulatory review. Maintaining a chain of custody safeguards the integrity of evidence and supports transparency if legal scrutiny arises later.

Time is a double-edged sword in fact gathering. While rapidity is essential to support timely disclosure and mitigation, rushing can lead to gaps or inaccurate conclusions. Conversely, excessive delay risks losing vital information as memories fade, records are overwritten, or witnesses become unavailable. Developing a structured yet flexible process that enables swift but thorough assessment is therefore a cornerstone of good practice. A well-designed incident reporting protocol, coupled with training and clear roles, empowers healthcare teams to balance speed with accuracy effectively.

Once initial data is collected, synthesising the information into a coherent incident narrative requires careful analysis. Patterns, contradictions, and contributory factors must be teased out to differentiate patient-specific issues from systemic failures. This stage often reveals the complexity of healthcare delivery, where multiple elements interplay, including staffing levels, workflows, environmental factors, and human behaviours converge in ways that rarely lend themselves to simplistic explanations. A comprehensive assessment embraces this complexity rather than seeking quick fixes, laying the groundwork for meaningful learning and improvement.

Effective fact-gathering also includes identifying all parties who need to be notified immediately, both internally and externally. Within healthcare organisations, seamless communication channels must be activated to engage clinical leaders, risk management teams, and patient safety officers. Externally, there may be requirements to inform regulators, legal advisors, or patient support services, depending on the nature and severity of the incident. Early notification ensures that resources can be mobilised and that subsequent actions, investigations, disclosures, or support mechanisms are coordinated rather than siloed. This coordination is essential to uphold the principles of candour and ensure consistency in messaging.

The psychological and emotional landscape during fact gathering cannot be overlooked. Both healthcare professionals involved in the incident and patients or their families are likely to be experiencing distress, anxiety, or even shock. Engaging with witnesses or colleagues soon after an event demands sensitivity to their emotional state while maintaining professional objectivity. Similarly, fact gathering must be conducted with due respect for patient dignity, privacy, and confidentiality. Skilled communication at this juncture, even when the focus is primarily on information collection, helps to foster an atmosphere of respect and compassion.

In some cases, fact-gathering must extend beyond the immediate team to include multidisciplinary input, especially when an incident reflects or reveals systemic issues. Engaging hospital risk managers, quality improvement specialists, infection control experts, or legal counsel as early partners can expedite the identification of broader contributing factors and ensure compliance with institutional policies. Their expertise can also guide the prioritisation of subsequent steps and highlight potential legal or ethical concerns that may arise during disclosure.

Documenting the fact-finding process meticulously, with timestamps and a clear record of sources and observations, is paramount. This documentation will form part of the official incident report and may be referenced in subsequent investigations, regulatory reviews, or legal proceedings. Well-structured records allow for transparency and accountability, demonstrating the healthcare professional's commitment to responsible practice. They also support reflective learning, enabling teams to assess not just what went wrong but also how the fact-gathering and initial response might be improved.

Preparation can substantially ease the burden of fact gathering when incidents occur. Healthcare organisations that invest in training staff in effective incident assessment techniques and that provide clear protocols and resources cultivate readiness and confidence. Simulation exercises that replicate the realities of real-world harm events foster familiarity with key steps, helping mitigate the inherent stress and complexity of such situations. Indeed, the development of a culture that normalises fact-gathering as a core component of the duty of candour helps embed transparency as a routine aspect of care rather than an exceptional or feared practice.

Finally, fact gathering is not a solitary endeavour; it is a collective responsibility that benefits from mutual support, shared expertise, and a common ethical commitment to patient safety and truthfulness. Coordinating efforts, whether through formal incident response teams or ad hoc collaboration, enhances the depth and reliability of the information collected. The ultimate purpose is clear: to understand fully what has happened, to communicate honestly with patients and families, and to use that knowledge to prevent recurrence. Fact-gathering and incident assessment, conducted promptly and thoroughly, transform difficult moments into opportunities for healing, learning, and systemic advancement in the pursuit of safer healthcare.

Notifying Internal Teams

In the delicate moments immediately following an adverse event, one of the most critical actions healthcare professionals must take is to promptly and thoughtfully notify internal teams. This step, while often perceived as an administrative formality, is in truth a cornerstone of effective incident management. Alerting managers and support staff rapidly and with precision not only helps to contain potential harm but also establishes the foundation for a transparent and coordinated response. These notifications, handled with sensitivity and urgency, enable the healthcare organisation to align its resources, deploy support mechanisms for patients and staff alike, and fulfil the ethical responsibility inherent in the duty of candour.

As soon as a significant incident is recognised, the urgency lies not only in securing the patient's immediate safety but equally in ensuring that the right people within the organisation are made aware, so that decisions and support can be mobilised expediently. The initial notification must be conveyed with clarity and without delay, striking a balance between expeditiousness and accuracy. This initial communication is rarely the full story; instead, it is a carefully calibrated alert that opens channels for further information gathering and collaboration. Managers, clinical leads, risk officers, and administrative support staff all play distinct but interlocking roles in managing the incident pathway. In practice, the healthcare professional who first identifies the event often bears responsibility for making the initial call or sending the first communication, setting the tone for subsequent actions. They must do so while controlling their own emotional response and maintaining professionalism, an imperative that calls for both preparation and empathy.

One of the most common pitfalls in this early notification phase is hesitancy born of fear of blame, repercussions, or reputational damage to oneself or the institution. However, the duty of candour requires healthcare workers to overcome these anxieties and prioritise patient well-being and organisational learning. Transparency at the outset encourages a culture in which issues are addressed promptly and openly, rather than suppressed or overlooked. It is worth remembering that internal reporting structures, established protocols, and chain-of-command communications exist precisely to support clinicians and staff in managing such situations effectively. A well-timed notification triggers the activation of resources such as incident response teams, patient safety officers, and counselling services. It also allows leadership to prepare for the more public-facing tasks of communicating with patients, families, or regulatory bodies.

When considering whom to notify internally, it is important to understand the organisational hierarchy and responsibility matrix, which will vary depending on the healthcare setting's size, speciality, and governance model. Typically, the immediate line manager or supervisor of the involved healthcare professional constitutes the first point of contact. This individual often acts as an intermediary between frontline staff and senior management or risk teams, helping to coordinate the response and maintain oversight. Healthcare managers possess the authority and experience to prioritise actions, allocate resources swiftly, and guide staff during an emotionally charged and operationally complex time. Managers also bear the ethical and professional duty to ensure appropriate follow-through, safeguarding the interests of patients and the institution alike.

Simultaneously, it is essential to inform the organisation's risk management or patient safety department. These specialised teams take a systematic view, connecting the dots across incidents, tracking trends, and facilitating comprehensive root cause analyses. They have expertise in navigating the multifaceted regulatory landscape and provide clinicians and managers with crucial advice on legal implications and documentation standards. By engaging risk managers early, healthcare professionals benefit from coordinated oversight that can mitigate further harm and protect the quality of care. Support from these dedicated teams reassures staff and contributes to a culture where learning from errors is normalised rather than stigmatised.

Alongside managerial and risk personnel, notifying relevant support staff such as clinical governance advisors, legal counsel, and communications teams can provide a broader scaffold around the incident. Clinical governance advisors often serve as lynchpins between clinical operations and organisational policies, ensuring that responses align with best practices and regulatory requirements. They may facilitate the initiation of formal investigations, audits, or peer reviews that underpin learning and improvement. Legal advisors, while not always engaged immediately, become critical when the incident involves potential litigation risks or compliance questions. Early engagement helps to frame communications in a way that is both transparent and protects professional and institutional integrity. Internal communications teams prepare to handle any external media inquiries and support messaging that respects confidentiality while maintaining openness. Engaging them early preserves a unified and responsible organisational voice.

The method and content of notification to internal teams must be tailored carefully to the urgency and nature of the incident without compromising clarity or sensitivity. In many healthcare settings, the preferred channel may be a direct phone call or face-to-face briefing, emphasising the gravity and personal responsibility involved. Texts or emails serve as supplementary tools but can risk misunderstandings or perceived detachment if relied upon exclusively. The content should provide a concise yet factual description of what has occurred, the immediate status of the patient, and any known contributing factors or risks. Including the steps already taken to secure safety demonstrates proactive management and reassures recipients that the incident is under control. It is equally important to avoid speculation or assigning blame at this early stage, focusing instead on transparent information sharing and prompt escalation.

Healthcare organisations often have predefined incident reporting systems, sometimes digitised, designed to capture key information in a structured format. The initial notification should complement, not replace, these formal reports. Combining swift verbal or written alerts with thorough documentation ensures that circulating awareness is joined by an accurate record for future reference and analysis. Good documentation reflects clarity, objectivity, and chronological details, creating a reliable foundation for investigations and disclosures. Ensuring that internal teams receive both the immediate alert and subsequent reports aids in developing a comprehensive understanding of the event, necessary for delivering the duty of candour appropriately to patients and families.

An often-underappreciated aspect of internal notification is the provision of emotional and professional support to the healthcare staff involved. Incidents that trigger the duty of candour can exact a heavy psychological toll, leading to feelings of guilt, shame, and anxiety about repercussions. Managers receiving early notification are entrusted not only with coordinating operational responses but also with recognising and addressing the needs of their team members. Prompt engagement enables the offering of debriefing sessions, peer support, or referrals to counselling services. This support helps to preserve morale, prevent burnout, and cultivate a culture where transparency is linked to mutual care rather than punishment. Staff must understand that reporting an incident and participating in the duty of candour process is an ethical obligation free from blame, fostering resilience and continued professional development.

To optimise internal notification processes, healthcare organisations benefit from regular training and simulation exercises that familiarise staff with protocols and communication expectations. When frontline professionals and managers practice real-time incident alerts through role-play or scenario-based drills, they become less daunted by the prospect of reporting. Clear guidelines that specify who to contact, how to document, and what information to relay empower staff to act swiftly and confidently. Training should emphasise the human elements of empathy, tone, and timing, ensuring that notifications respect the dignity of all involved. Simultaneously, review mechanisms that assess how well notifications were conducted after an incident contribute to continuous improvement, closing the feedback loop and refining organisational preparedness.

In navigating the complexities of internal notifications, healthcare professionals must also consider the phenomenon of information overload during critical incidents. An overly broad disclosure of incident details to irrelevant parties can cause confusion, breach confidentiality, or unnecessarily escalate worry. Conversely, failing to inform key personnel can result in fragmented responses and missed opportunities for prompt intervention. Therefore, notification strategies must be deliberate and judicious, adhering to principles of need-to-know balance with an eye towards operational accountability. This balance ensures that the response is neither paralysed by indecision nor compromised by disorganisation, ultimately fortifying patient safety and trust.

Furthermore, in complex organisations that span multiple sites or specialties, interdepartmental communication requires careful coordination. Notifying managers and staff within the immediate clinical area is only the first layer; broader organisational awareness may be necessary if the incident impacts systemic processes or involves cross-disciplinary teams. In such contexts, internal notification cascades structured, tiered communication pathways can be invaluable tools. These cascades ensure that information flows up through management levels efficiently while also descending to staff who will be involved in remediation efforts. Ensuring that such systems are up-to-date and well-understood minimises delays and errors in information sharing.

The goal of internal notification transcends mere administrative compliance; it is fundamentally about creating the conditions under which honesty, support, and resolution can emerge. By alerting managers and support staff with timely, accurate, and considerate communications, healthcare professionals initiate a collaborative process that acknowledges harm, seeks understanding, and commits to improvement. This process embodies the spirit of the duty of candour by fostering an environment where difficult truths are confronted not with fear or defensiveness, but with courage and compassion.

In summary, the notification of internal teams after an adverse event is an intricate and indispensable element of the duty of candour. It requires healthcare professionals to respond promptly and sensitively, communicating key information to managers, risk officers, and support personnel in a manner that is clear, factual, and respectful. This notification serves as the gateway to coordinated incident management, patient safety interventions, emotional support for staff, and ultimately transparent disclosure to patients and families. Organisations that cultivate robust internal notification protocols and train their teams accordingly empower their staff to navigate these challenging moments confidently and competently, reinforcing a culture of openness that benefits all stakeholders. The responsibility to notify internal teams is not simply a task to be completed but a vital gesture of the collaborative, trustworthy, and patient-centred ethos at the heart of modern healthcare.

Communicating with Patients and Families: What to Say and How to Say It

Preparing for the Conversation

Preparing for the conversation about an adverse event with a patient or their family is a delicate, weighty task that demands both careful planning and a thoughtful mindset. It is not merely about the content of what will be shared but also profoundly about how, when, and where the disclosure takes place, with an unwavering commitment to honesty and empathy. At its core, preparation involves constructing a framework that balances transparency with compassion, alongside a readiness to engage authentically with the often raw and intense emotions that inevitably arise. Recognising the gravity of this moment for all parties involved underscores the necessity for healthcare professionals to approach disclosure conversations with a blend of professionalism, empathy, and humanity.

The first essential step is selecting a setting conducive to a respectful, open dialogue where the patient or family feels safe and supported. This means opting for a private, quiet space free from interruptions and distractions, where the focus can remain entirely on the conversation. Such an environment not only reduces discomfort but signals to the patient and family that their experience and feelings are valued. The physical space should be comfortable, perhaps with seating arranged to promote eye contact and intimacy rather than a hierarchical dynamic. Avoid clinical settings that feel stark or impersonal; instead, choose a room that allows warmth to permeate the interaction, thereby easing anxiety and fostering trust. Scheduling the conversation at a time when the relevant healthcare team members can be present or promptly available also supports a seamless and coherent disclosure, reassuring the patient or family that the healthcare system stands united in addressing what has occurred.

Timing is equally critical and requires a sensitive, strategic approach. Ideally, disclosure should happen as soon as reasonably possible once the essential facts have been gathered and understood, delaying for too long risks eroding trust and causing additional distress. However, rushing prematurely without clarity or full preparedness can lead to confusion or unintended miscommunication. Preparing yourself to strike this balance involves gathering as much accurate information as possible prior to the conversation, while also acknowledging any ongoing uncertainties. Transparency about what is known and unknown at this stage can build credibility and demonstrate integrity, rather than suggest evasiveness. Additionally, understanding the patient's or family's emotional and cognitive readiness will guide timing decisions; if they are currently overwhelmed or engaged in other distressing news, it may be necessary to pause briefly to allow them space before approaching the disclosure.

Choosing the right language to use during the conversation demands profound care and forethought. It is essential to communicate in simple, clear terms that avoid jargon and technical complexity, which may alienate or confuse listeners. The goal is to be direct and truthful without unnecessarily escalating fear or guilt. For example, instead of saying, "there was an adverse event," an explanation along the lines of, "something happened during your care that we believe caused you harm," is more tangible and personal. Words carry immense power, so each phrase should be carefully considered for its potential impact on feelings of blame, shame, or hope. This also includes framing discussions to avoid defensiveness; focusing on the event and its effects, rather than attributing fault without clear evidence, helps maintain an atmosphere conducive to healing. Using language that conveys remorse, compassion, and a genuine desire to resolve the incident and learn from it builds bridges rather than walls during this difficult exchange.

Parallel to preparing language is the essential work of self-regulation and emotional preparation as a healthcare professional. Approaching these conversations confidently requires practitioners to manage their own emotions. This means acknowledging feelings of guilt, fear, or anxiety privately beforehand, so that during the disclosure, the focus can remain steadfastly on the patient and family without awkwardness or distraction. Practising mindfulness techniques or engaging in peer support or supervision in advance can fortify emotional resilience, allowing the clinician to remain calm and empathetic. It is important to remember that conveying sincerity does not require suppressing feelings but channelling them appropriately to reflect humanity and empathy. When professionals prepare mentally to meet patient distress with steady receptiveness and openness, the entire encounter gains authenticity and meaning. Managing one's body language, ensuring a relaxed posture, steady eye contact, and a gentle tone, reinforces calmness and compassion in the dialogue, reducing the potential for unintended signals of defensiveness or detachment.

Clinicians should anticipate that difficult questions will arise and mentally rehearse how to respond honestly yet sensitively. Patients or families may ask why the incident happened, who is responsible, what will be done to prevent recurrence, or inquire about legal implications. It is vital not to evade these inquiries but to answer them truthfully to the best of one's knowledge, while setting realistic expectations if some answers remain uncertain. Practising responses ahead of time helps in avoiding jargon or overly technical explanations, replacing them with candid, clear communication. Where direct knowledge is lacking, it is acceptable and indeed advisable to acknowledge this and commit to providing updates as information becomes available. This approach not only upholds honesty but also models the transparency that underpins the duty of candour. It helps to consider the legal and institutional guidance around disclosure, ensuring that statements align with regulatory and organisational policies without compromising compassion or openness.

Maintaining trust throughout the conversation is paramount and depends largely on the attitude brought to the disclosure. Starting the discussion with an expression of empathy and, where appropriate, an apology can diffuse initial tension and speak volumes about the clinician's care. Apologies must be sincere, addressing the specific impact of the incident rather than offering generic or defensive apologies that may be perceived as insincere or evasive. For example, acknowledging the distress the patient or family must be feeling, expressing genuine sorrow for the harm caused, and affirming a commitment to support them moving forward helps to build rapport. Avoiding platitudes or minimising the incident demonstrates respect for the emotional reality of those affected. Moreover, professionals should be prepared to listen actively and validate feelings without rushing to move the conversation forward prematurely. Acknowledging silence and allowing spaces for emotional responses, including tears, anger, or shock, shows respect and patience, reinforcing trust even in moments of discomfort.

Another key aspect of preparation is coordinating with the wider healthcare team to ensure a unified approach to disclosure and subsequent actions. This involves clarifying roles: identifying who will lead the conversation, what roles support staff might play, and establishing agreed messaging to avoid conflicting information. Collaboration with the risk management and communications teams before the meeting may provide additional perspectives on phrasing, content, and how to handle potential media interest or legal questions. Such preparation signals to patients and families that the healthcare organisation is earnest in managing the event comprehensively and transparently. Internal alignment also extends to subsequent care plans and follow-up, ensuring that promises made during disclosure, such as additional support, further investigations, or updates, are fulfilled consistently and punctually.

Further depth in preparation includes reflecting on one's own values and motivations related to candour. Recognising that disclosure is not merely an obligation but an ethical commitment to respect patients' dignity and autonomy can shift the clinician's mindset from apprehension to responsibility and even privilege. This mental framing helps navigate the discomfort that often accompanies such conversations by anchoring disclosure in the broader purpose of trust-building and patient-centred care. It also opens space to embrace the inherent vulnerability of the moment, acknowledging that sharing difficult truths can promote healing and strengthen relational bonds rather than rupture them. As such, cultivating a compassionate and non-defensive internal narrative before the meeting is an invaluable component of readiness.

Practically, preparing for the conversation may also include rehearsing specific conversation scripts or prompts that guide the flow of dialogue. While rigidity must be avoided to maintain authenticity, having anchor points, such as how to begin, ways to transition between explaining facts and addressing emotions, and methods for concluding with steps forward, provides a helpful scaffold for confidence. Practitioners can balance rehearsed wording with responsive listening, adapting to the unique dynamics of each interaction. This practice helps mitigate fear of unknown reactions and builds a repertoire of language that seamlessly balances honesty, clarity, and compassion.

Attention to cultural competence and individual patient or family preferences is another critical preparatory layer. Recognising that people process and respond to difficult news differently based on cultural, spiritual, and personal backgrounds means that clinicians should tailor their approach accordingly. This may involve prior inquiry into preferred communication styles, language needs, or the presence of support persons. Ensuring access to interpreters or culturally appropriate resources signals respect and inclusivity. Being prepared to adapt the conversation to meet these needs improves understanding and fosters a connection that transcends mere information transmission.

Finally, clinicians should prepare not only for the initial disclosure but also for ongoing communication and continued support. This means setting the stage for open lines of communication after the conversation, ensuring that patients and families know whom to contact with further questions or concerns. Providing reassurance that the disclosure is not a one-time event but part of an ongoing commitment to transparency and care helps to sustain trust over time. Preparing follow-up documentation, contact details, and arrangements for psychological or social support, as needed, anticipates the needs that often arise after difficult conversations. Being proactive in this manner reflects a holistic understanding of the impact of harm and the role of disclosure in the broader healing process.

In summary, preparing for the disclosure conversation is a multifaceted endeavour that requires healthcare professionals to synchronise practical arrangements, cultivate a mindful, empathetic mindset, use clear, compassionate language, foster teamwork, and demonstrate cultural sensitivity. It demands that clinicians prepare emotionally, intellectually, and logistically to engage in a dialogue that is not only truthful about the harm done but also unwaveringly compassionate and supportive. Through such preparation, these difficult conversations can transform from moments of fear and uncertainty into profound opportunities for connection, learning, and renewed trust, ultimately advancing the goal of a transparent and patient-centred healthcare environment.

Delivering Clear and Compassionate Messages

Delivering clear and compassionate messages in the wake of an adverse healthcare event is a delicate and profoundly sensitive task. It requires more than just conveying facts; it involves an intricate blend of emotional intelligence, timing, cultural awareness, and interpersonal skills to ensure that the communication is not only understood but also received in a way that fosters trust, healing, and mutual respect. The moment when a healthcare professional must share difficult news about a complication, error, or harm can shape the entire patient and family experience. Done well, it reinforces the therapeutic alliance, supports patient autonomy, and sets the stage for constructive dialogue moving forward. Done poorly, it compounds distress, breeds mistrust and may hinder the very goals of safety and transparency that the duty of candour embodies.

Choosing the appropriate language lies at the heart of this endeavour. Medical terminology, while precise in clinical settings, often becomes a barrier rather than a bridge when communicating with patients and families who are unfamiliar with its nuances. The challenge is to translate complex concepts into accessible, jargon-free language without sounding patronising or vague. A compassionate communicator selects words that are straightforward and concrete, avoiding euphemisms or ambiguous phrases that may obscure understanding or cause confusion. For example, rather than saying "There was a complication during your procedure," explaining gently, "During your operation, something didn't go as expected, and I want to explain what happened," provides clarity while preparing the listener for the seriousness of the information. The tone should be calm, steady, and free from overt professional detachment; warmth conveyed through vocal inflexions and word choice helps humanise the dialogue and acknowledge the patient's vulnerability.

Equally important is the timing of these conversations. There is an instinct to delay or defer difficult disclosures to shield patients and families from distress or to buy time for complete information gathering. While well-intentioned, postponing conversations risks eroding trust and may fuel suspicion or anxiety as patients sense something is being withheld. The duty of candour encourages timely disclosure, recognising that early, honest conversations, even when all details are unknown, demonstrate respect and openness. This means preparing for the discussion as soon as feasible, arranging a private setting, and ensuring that key members of the care team are available to provide support and continuity. Prompt engagement allows the healthcare provider to frame the narrative honestly, acknowledge uncertainty, and commit to ongoing communication. It also provides patients and families the dignity of facing the reality with proactive support rather than reactive crisis management.

Setting the right environment for disclosure conversations profoundly affects their tone and outcome. Privacy, comfort, and minimal interruptions are essential. Conversations should occur in a quiet room where patients and families feel physically safe, at ease, and able to focus without distraction. The clinician should sit at eye level, facing the patient to foster connection, avoid barriers such as desks or computer screens that create physical and psychological distance, and use open body language that signals attentiveness and empathy. Preparing the room by ensuring tissues are available, water is readily available, and the seating arrangement promotes calm dialogue can subtly reassure recipients. Lighting should be warm rather than harsh, and noise should be reduced to prevent unnecessary interruptions. All efforts coalesce in an environment that signals respect and care, removing physical clutter to allow emotional and conversational space.

Managing emotions, both those of the patient or family and the clinician, is perhaps one of the most challenging aspects of delivering clear and compassionate messages. The disclosure of harm often unleashes a torrent of feelings: fear, anger, confusion, sadness, and sometimes blame. Healthcare professionals must cultivate patience, active listening, and emotional resilience in these moments. Responses to emotional expressions should be validating rather than dismissive. For instance, when a parent expresses anger at a perceived error, a response such as "I can hear how upset this is making you, and that feeling is completely understandable," acknowledges their pain without defensiveness or minimisation. Silence, when appropriate, can be a powerful tool that allows space for grieving or reflection. Simultaneously, clinicians must manage their own feelings of vulnerability, guilt, or fear of repercussions; through training, peer support, and self-awareness, they can maintain composure that reassures recipients and facilitates constructive engagement.

Answering difficult questions during disclosure demands honesty balanced with sensitivity. Patients and families may seek explanations about how and why the harm occurred, what could have been done differently, and what steps will be taken to prevent recurrence. Being direct, eschewing evasiveness, affirms respect for their need to understand. When facts are still being determined, it is appropriate to acknowledge this uncertainty openly: "We are still reviewing the events, and I will share everything we learn with you as soon as possible." Avoiding speculation and sticking to verified information helps maintain credibility. Equally, recognising when questions arise from emotional distress rather than factual curiosity allows the clinician to address underlying fears and needs for reassurance. It is also vital to tackle misconceptions gently and correct misinformation to guide future expectations. Ensuring that communication flows bidirectionally, where patients feel heard, and their inquiries are addressed sincerely, strengthens the alliance.

Maintaining trust through honesty and compassion is the cornerstone of effective duty of candour practice. Trust is fragile, often shaken by harm or perceived opacity in communication. Healthcare professionals rebuild this trust by consistently demonstrating openness, admitting shortcomings without defensiveness, and prioritising the patient's well-being over self-interest. Transparency about what is known, what remains to be discovered, and what is being done to investigate and rectify the issue conveys a commitment to accountability. Compassion complements honesty by conveying genuine concern, empathy, and respect for the person behind the patient status. Communicating not only the facts but also the values driving the response, including a pledge to improve and prevent future harm, helps solidify trust. Moreover, following through on promises made during disclosure conversations, such as arranging further meetings, providing written summaries, or facilitating additional support, is critical to sustaining confidence.

Crafting these conversations also involves an acute awareness of cultural, social, and individual differences that shape how information is received and processed. What constitutes compassionate communication in one cultural context may diverge sharply in another; some patients may value bluntness and directness, while others expect a more nuanced and deferential approach. Being attuned to these preferences through cultural competence training, respectful inquiry, and mindful observation enables clinicians to tailor messages effectively. For example, understanding that some families may prefer all decision-makers to be present or require interpreters to grasp the conversation fully enhances inclusivity and comprehension. Likewise, recognition of differing health literacy levels guides adjustments to language complexity. Implementing these adaptations ensures that disclosure is not only transparent but also accessible and respectful.

An often overlooked yet critical component is preparing for and managing the flow of the conversation itself. Starting with an introduction that frames the purpose, respectfully acknowledges the gravity of the situation, and expresses an intent to be open sets a tone of honesty and care. Leading with a clear statement such as "I want to talk about what happened during your care because you deserve to know the truth" establishes transparency up front. Allowing the patient or family first to express their understanding or concerns provides essential insight into their current emotional and cognitive state and guides the subsequent discourse. Following this, explaining the known facts, the potential implications, and the immediate next steps in plain language allows shared understanding. Throughout, checking in on the listener's reactions and inviting questions or clarifications helps maintain engagement and avoid misunderstandings. Concluding with reassurance about ongoing support and availability underscores the continued care relationship.

Effective communication in this context also requires recognition of the power dynamics inherent in healthcare settings and a striving to equalise interactions as much as possible. Patients and families may feel vulnerable or intimidated by medical authority, particularly when unexpected harm has occurred. Acknowledging this imbalance through empathetic dialogue, fostering a sense of partnership, and encouraging active participation in decisions about investigations or remedial actions empowers them. Statements such as "We want to work with you to learn what went wrong and how we can improve" position the patient or family as collaborators rather than passive recipients of information. This approach promotes a shared journey toward healing and system improvement.

Using non-verbal communication effectively enhances the message's clarity and compassion. Maintaining eye contact, nodding affirmatively, and mirroring the patient's or family's emotional tone can provide unspoken comfort and reinforce attentive listening. Avoiding distracting gestures, such as checking a watch or a computer screen, keeps the focus on the person conversing, signalling that their words and feelings are important. Gentle tone modulation avoids the perception of clinical detachment. When tears or visible distress occur, allowing the space for these expressions without urgency to move on respects the emotive process, humanising the interaction.

There will be instances where multiple professionals participate in the disclosure conversation, such as a lead clinician accompanied by a nurse, social worker, or patient liaison. Coordination among team members beforehand about roles, messaging, and responsibilities ensures consistency and avoids mixed messages that can undermine trust. It also provides a support network for both the patient and clinician, contributing to a comprehensive approach that addresses medical, emotional, and logistical considerations.

The inclusion of an apology, when appropriate, forms a cornerstone of compassionate disclosure. Understanding how to express regret without implying automatic legal liability is essential to avoid fear-driven silence. Phrases that communicate sorrow for the suffering or distress caused, rather than specific admissions of fault before a full investigation, can ease patients' hurt and foster reconciliation. For example, saying "I am deeply sorry that this happened to you and that you experienced harm under our care" acknowledges human frailty and institutional responsibility without risking premature legal exposure. This delicate balance requires skill and often institutional guidance to navigate safely.

Lastly, it is important to remember that delivering clear and compassionate messages is not a one-time event but rather part of an ongoing dialogue. The initial disclosure conversation opens the door but does not close it. Patients and families may require follow-up meetings to absorb information, ask new questions, or express emerging feelings. Offering continuing availability helps maintain openness and reinforces commitment to transparency. Documenting these conversations carefully, while respecting the privacy and dignity of those involved, supports organisational learning and accountability without compromising the personalised nature of each interaction.

In summary, the art of delivering clear and compassionate messages after harm in healthcare is both a science and a deeply human practice. It demands deliberate attention to language, timing, setting, emotional management, transparency, and cultural empathy. By continuously honing these communication skills, healthcare professionals can transform difficult encounters into opportunities for healing, learning, and renewed trust. Such mastery not only fulfils the duty of candour but also embodies the core values of compassionate, patient-centred care.

Managing Emotional Responses

In the delicate and often distressing moments following an adverse event in healthcare, one of the most profound challenges faced by clinicians, patients, and families alike is the management of emotional responses. These encounters are inherently charged with vulnerability, hurt, fear, and sometimes anger, making open communication deeply complex. The imperative for healthcare professionals is not only to provide factual clarity but to do so in a manner that honours and supports the emotional landscapes of all parties involved. The essence of managing emotional responses in the context of duty of candour is rooted in empathy, an active, conscious engagement with the feelings of others and in maintaining a steady compass of compassion that guides every interaction.

For patients and families, the experience of harm or unexpected outcomes shatters the trust and safety they have invested in their healthcare providers. Their emotions can oscillate rapidly between confusion, grief, frustration, and anxiety. These responses are natural reactions to uncertainty and perceived loss of control, and recognising this emotional turmoil is a vital first step for clinicians preparing to undertake disclosure conversations. Acknowledgement of feelings must be woven seamlessly into communication, not merely as a courteous preamble but as an essential aspect of healing. When a healthcare professional sincerely validates the emotional reality of a patient or family member, it can diffuse defensiveness and open a channel for honest dialogue. Statements gently affirming the patient's distress, such as "I can see this is very upsetting for you" or "It's entirely understandable to feel angry or confused right now", signal that the professional is present with them in the experience, not apart from it. This empathetic presence itself is a powerful therapeutic tool.

Clinicians, however, are no strangers to the emotional burden that accompanies adverse events. Feelings of guilt, shame, fear of blame, and personal sorrow can weigh heavily, often compounded by the inherent stress of clinical responsibilities. Emotional responses from clinicians, if unacknowledged, can impede open communication and lead to guarded or defensive behaviour. It is vital that healthcare professionals cultivate self-awareness of their own feelings and develop strategies to regulate them, remaining authentic and supportive in interactions. Self-reflection and, where possible, peer support or supervision can help clinicians untangle personal emotions from the patient's needs at the moment of disclosure. Managing one's own emotional response does not mean suppressing feelings but rather channelling them so that they enhance the capacity for compassionate honesty instead of triggering avoidance or denial.

Choosing the appropriate time and setting for these conversations plays a foundational role in emotional management. The environment must offer privacy and comfort, allowing all parties to express their feelings freely without fear of interruption or exposure. While the urgency for disclosure should not be delayed unnecessarily, rushed or public disclosures often exacerbate distress and can generate feelings of abandonment or disrespect. Gentle pacing, allowing space for silence or tears, and ensuring adequate time not just for delivering information but also for listening can transform a difficult disclosure into a moment of connection and trust-building. Healthcare leaders have a responsibility to support clinicians by providing suitable spaces and realistic schedules that respect the emotional demands of this work.

Language choice is another crucial element in navigating emotional responses. Words carry immense weight, especially in moments of heightened sensitivity. Healthcare professionals must strive for clarity without clinical coldness, honesty without abruptness, and compassion without pity. Avoiding jargon or evasive language prevents confusion and mistrust, but bluntness without empathy can deepen wounds. For instance, instead of saying "There was a complication," a more sensitive phrasing might be, "During your treatment, something unexpected happened that affected your recovery." This framing acknowledges the event candidly, while gentle framing cushions the impact. Moreover, anticipatory guidance, preparing patients and families for the nature of the conversation ahead, can reduce shock and emotional overwhelm. Introducing discussions with phrases like "I want to talk with you about what happened and answer any questions you might have" sets a collaborative tone that respects patient autonomy and emotional readiness.

During the conversation, actively listening is as important as what is said. Patients and families will express a wide range of emotions, sometimes through tears, silence, or anger, and the clinician's response should be attuned to these cues without rushing to fill every pause or silence. This capacity to hold space for grief or frustration is a testament to genuine care and validation. When confronted with difficult questions, which inevitably arise, honesty must be tempered with an understanding of the emotional weight behind those inquiries. It is acceptable to acknowledge when information is not yet available, and to commit transparently to ongoing communication, rather than offering premature or speculative answers. Such openness sustains trust even amid uncertainty.

Supporting patients and families extends beyond the initial conversation. For some, the period following disclosure is laden with ongoing emotional distress and requires signposting to additional resources, such as counselling services, patient advocates, or support groups. Clinicians should be mindful not to leave families feeling isolated after difficult news; repeated offers of support and availability demonstrate a commitment to their well-being beyond the technical repair of a clinical error. Likewise, allowing families to express their needs and preferences for follow-up communication fosters a sense of control and partnership in their own care pathway.

From the clinician's perspective, access to psychological support and reflective practice forums is essential to prevent burnout and compassion fatigue, which can erode the ability to manage emotions professionally. Organisations that actively prioritise the emotional wellness of their staff create environments where candour flourishes. The culture of openness becomes sustainable only when clinicians feel safe, not just legally but emotionally, to engage in these difficult conversations. Leaders can foster this by modelling vulnerability and normalising discussions about the emotional impact of adverse events.

In conclusion, the journey of managing emotional responses in the duty of candour process demands a delicate balancing act: clinicians must courageously face their own feelings and anxieties while placing the lived experience of patients and families at the heart of each interaction. Every disclosure conversation is a unique encounter shaped by human emotion, and it requires the clinician to embody patience, empathy, and transparency with profound skill. When this is done thoughtfully, what begins as a painful moment can evolve into a foundational experience of trust and mutual respect. Such moments, though difficult, have the power to heal wounds deeper than physical harm, restoring faith in the healthcare relationship and fostering a culture where openness and integrity are the cornerstones of care.

Saying Sorry: Timing, Content and Professional Boundaries

The Role of Apology in Healing

In the intricate interplay of healthcare interactions, where trust is both fragile and invaluable, the act of apology serves as a profound catalyst for healing, a gesture that transcends the mere acknowledgement of error to affirm humanity, empathy, and accountability in the face of harm. When adverse events occur, the aftermath often leaves patients and their families enveloped in confusion, fear, and grief, emotions that demand more than clinical explanations or procedural responses. A sincere apology breaks through these barriers, restoring a connection that honours the patient's experience and validates their feelings. It is within this delicate moment that healthcare professionals can bridge the chasm wrought by unintended harm, transforming a narrative of loss and mistrust into one of compassion, respect, and genuine concern. The significance of apology in this context extends beyond a customary or procedural act; it fulfils a moral and relational imperative at the very heart of patient-centred care.

Understanding when to offer an apology requires not only legal and institutional awareness but, importantly, an attuned sense of the patient's needs and the context of the incident. Apologies are not reserved solely for clear-cut cases of fault or negligence; rather, they are appropriate whenever a patient experiences harm linked to healthcare delivery, regardless of the cause. This distinction is essential, as an apology does not automatically equate to an admission of liability but rather serves as a means of expressing empathy and regret for the suffering endured. Delaying or withholding an apology can exacerbate the patient's distress, eroding trust further and potentially hindering healing. Promptness in offering an apology signals openness and respect, demonstrating that the healthcare professional acknowledges the patient's experience and is committed to transparency. This initial step often marks the beginning of constructive dialogue that can pave the way for shared understanding and mutual respect, even amidst difficult circumstances.

The content of an effective apology demands careful articulation, a balancing act that marries candidness with sensitivity. At its core, an apology should convey genuine regret for the impact the incident has had on the patient and their loved ones, affirming that their pain is recognised and taken seriously. It must avoid vague platitudes that may seem dismissive while steering clear of language that might unintentionally imply culpability without due process. A well-crafted apology carefully addresses the emotional, informational, and relational dimensions: it succinctly acknowledges what happened, expresses sincere sorrow, and outlines the steps being taken to investigate and address the issue. Transparency about uncertainties or ongoing inquiries can further consolidate trust by demonstrating honesty, even in the face of incomplete information. The apology should also emphasise the healthcare professional's commitment to learning from the event, reinforcing that the patient's experience is not just an unfortunate mishap, but a critical impetus for improvement.

Legal considerations play a nuanced role in shaping how apologies are delivered in healthcare settings. Various jurisdictions interpret the legal ramifications of apologetic statements differently, with some offering protections that prevent an apology from being used as evidence of liability, while others remain cautious about such disclosures. Healthcare professionals must, therefore, be acutely aware of their local legal frameworks and institutional policies, balancing the ethical obligation to be honest and compassionate with the need to safeguard themselves and their organisations from undue legal jeopardy. This often means that apologies are framed carefully to express empathy and regret without explicitly admitting fault or error. The phrasing becomes crucial; words like "I am sorry that you have suffered" or "I regret what happened" focus on the emotional impact rather than on legal admission. Engaging with legal advisors and risk management teams helps professionals navigate this complex territory, ensuring that apologies fulfil their healing purpose without compromising legal or professional standing.

Maintaining professional boundaries in the apology is equally vital, as it ensures that the communication remains respectful, focused, and appropriate to the clinical relationship. While empathy is paramount, it must be expressed in a way that supports healing and restoration without crossing into territory that might confuse roles or expectations. For example, healthcare professionals should avoid making promises they cannot keep or engaging in behaviour that might be interpreted as personal liability beyond institutional responsibility. The apology should centre on the patient's experience and the shared objective of addressing harm and preventing recurrence, rather than on the clinician's personal emotional responses. This professional detachment does not diminish the sincerity of the apology; rather, it grounds the interaction in trustworthiness, clarity, and mutual respect. The intention is always to foster a therapeutic alliance, even amid difficulty, while preserving the patient's dignity and autonomy and upholding the healthcare provider's integrity.

Extensive research and countless narratives from patients and clinicians alike underscore the transformative power of apology in healthcare. Patients who receive timely, honest, and compassionate apologies are more likely to experience emotional closure, subsequently trust the healthcare system, and participate actively in their ongoing care. Furthermore, transparent disclosure, coupled with an apology, reduces litigation risk and facilitates reconciliation, providing a platform for dialogue that focuses on prevention and improvement rather than blame. For healthcare professionals, embracing apology nurtures a culture of openness and continuous learning, reducing the isolation and fear that often accompany adverse events. It empowers individuals and organisations to confront mistakes constructively, cultivating resilience and fostering safer care environments. In this way, apology is not a sign of weakness or failure but a demonstration of professional courage and ethical commitment.

Within many healthcare settings, the practice of apology encounters cultural and systemic challenges. Fear of repercussions, lack of training, or uncertainty about how to navigate complex emotional and legal landscapes can deter professionals from engaging openly. This reticence, however, often perpetuates the silence and suspicion that further harms patients. Institutional leadership plays a crucial role in normalising the duty of candour and supporting clinicians to apologise effectively and confidently. Providing education, clear policies, and emotional support equips healthcare workers with the skills and reassurance necessary to fulfil this vital component of care. Moreover, fostering an environment where apology is seen as a shared responsibility rather than an individual burden mitigates the stigma surrounding error disclosure. Over time, such cultural shifts pave the way for more authentic and healing interactions between clinicians and patients, reinforcing the social contract at the heart of healthcare.

Ultimately, the role of apology in healing within healthcare is a testament to the profession's core values of compassion, respect, and integrity. It embodies a commitment to truthfulness and kindness, acknowledging the profound vulnerability patients experience when care does not proceed as expected. By embracing apology not simply as a ceremonial gesture but as a meaningful, deliberate act of connection, healthcare professionals affirm their dedication to patient welfare beyond technical expertise. Each apology, when delivered with humility and care, becomes a seed of hope that nurtures trust, mends relationships, and inspires continual improvement. This transformative potential elevates the duty of candour from a legal or procedural obligation to a profound expression of the healing mission that lies at the heart of medicine and nursing. In this light, apology is not only about addressing what went wrong but about reaffirming what healthcare is ultimately about: the dignity, safety, and well-being of every patient entrusted to our care.

Crafting an Appropriate Apology

Apologising in the aftermath of an adverse event holds profound significance that extends far beyond mere words. An apology becomes a bridge, a vital connection that can restore fractured trust, soothe raw emotions, and affirm a shared humanity between healthcare professionals and those affected. Yet, the art of crafting an appropriate apology is not simply about saying "I'm sorry" and moving on; it demands careful thought, sensitivity, and a nuanced understanding of the legal, ethical, and relational boundaries within which it is delivered. What you say and just as importantly, what you avoid saying can profoundly influence the healing process, the restoration of dignity, and the ongoing nature of the professional relationship.

Timing sits at the heart of an apology's potency. It's essential to recognise that apologising too late can sometimes feel insincere or dismissive to patients and families who are already grappling with confusion, pain, and hurt. Conversely, an apology that is rushed, issued before all facts are clear, might unintentionally lock clinicians into positions of legal vulnerability or cause unnecessary distress through premature conclusions. The ideal moment for an apology is often soon after the incident, once initial clinical priorities have been met, and a preliminary understanding of the event's basic parameters is established. This allows the apology to resonate as both genuine and informed, avoiding the pitfalls of vagueness yet not slipping into blame or defensiveness. It is important to remember that the apology should never be deferred indefinitely; silence can be misinterpreted as evasion or indifference, deepening mistrust and pain.

When composing the apology itself, the language chosen should be clear, straightforward, and imbued with sincere empathy. Avoid medical jargon or overly complex explanations at this early juncture. Patients and families need acknowledgement of their experience in terms they can grasp, which honours their feelings and situates their suffering as real and important. An effective apology conveys genuine sorrow and regret for the harm caused, without necessarily attributing legal liability or fault. Saying "I am truly sorry that you have suffered harm during your care" is a powerful and carefully balanced example. It acknowledges the distress without prematurely dissecting the cause or the mechanics of the error. Importantly, the apology should not shift blame, minimise the impact, or use conditional language that can sound dismissive, such as "I'm sorry if you feel upset" or "I'm sorry but…" Such phrases risk invalidating the patient's reality and may cause confusion or further harm.

Balancing empathy while maintaining professional boundaries requires deliberate skill. The apology must convey compassion without overpromising or implying certainty about every detail of what happened, particularly when investigations or reviews are ongoing. This balance is crucial to maintain trust not only with patients and families but also within the wider healthcare team and legal frameworks. Expressing empathy means listening attentively to the emotions and concerns conveyed by the patient or family and reflecting understanding back, for example, "I can only imagine how difficult this has been for you." These words acknowledge the emotional impact without crossing into speculation or offering unfounded assurances.

Equally important is understanding what must be avoided in a formal apology to protect both patients' rights and clinicians' professional safety. An apology should never include overt language that admits legal liability or explicitly states fault, such as "I admit that I made a mistake" or "We were negligent." While honesty and openness are fundamental to the duty of candour, such statements can be misused in litigation or insurance claims, potentially complicating resolution for all parties. Instead, clinicians should focus on transparency about the facts as they are known without conjecture, reiterating the organisation's commitment to investigating the event thoroughly and to making amends where possible. This approach aligns with best practices and legal guidance in many jurisdictions, which increasingly recognise apologies as part of compassionate care rather than admissions of guilt.

The apology should also include a clear outline of the next steps. Patients and families need to know that their concerns are being taken seriously and that actions will be taken to understand and, if possible, rectify what happened. Statements such as "We will review your care carefully and share with you what we learn" help demonstrate accountability and a commitment to learning that can mitigate feelings of abandonment or helplessness. This forward-looking element of the apology embodies responsibility without implying fault, signalling a dedication to systemic improvement and prevention of recurrence. It transforms the apology from a simple expression of regret into a promise of partnership in healing and safety.

Moreover, verbal apologies should ideally be supported by written communication. This reinforces sincerity and provides patients and families with a tangible record of transparency and care. However, written apologies need to be crafted with equal care, ensuring they reflect the same principles of empathy, clarity, and careful wording outlined above. In settings where multiple members of the healthcare team may be involved, coordinating a unified message avoids confusion and demonstrates organisational coherence. It's often helpful for apologies to come from both the individual clinician caring for the patient and a representative of the organisation's leadership, illustrating that candour is embedded at all levels.

The interpersonal context in which the apology is delivered also influences its effectiveness. A face-to-face meeting, when feasible, offers the richest environment for communication, allowing for tone, body language, and immediate reciprocal dialogue. It conveys respect and openness, encouraging questions and emotional expression. When in-person meetings are initially impossible due to geographic distance, patient or family preference, or ongoing clinical care, alternatives such as video calls can approximate these interactions better than letters or phone calls alone. Regardless of format, the healthcare professional delivering the apology must be prepared, supported, and able to respond authentically. This may involve rehearsing phrasing, consulting with legal or communication experts, or involving multidisciplinary team members to ensure clarity and compassion.

Finally, the emotional labour clinicians undertake in offering apologies should not be underestimated. Apologising effectively requires humility, reflection, and courage, qualities that may be challenged by fear, guilt, and anxiety about repercussions. Healthcare organisations must therefore create environments in which professionals feel supported in engaging openly with patients and families. Training in communication skills, access to counselling and peer support, and clear organisational policies that protect and empower clinicians are indispensable. This culture of support makes it more likely that apologies will be delivered appropriately and authentically, serving their essential purpose in healing and accountability rather than becoming sources of further distress.

In summary, crafting an appropriate apology is a delicate balance between expressing sincere empathy and maintaining professional boundaries. It involves careful timing, clear and compassionate language, avoidance of admissions of legal liability, and a commitment to transparency and follow-up. When done well, apologies can be transformative, rebuilding trust in the face of harm, validating the experiences of patients and families, and fostering a culture of continuous learning and improvement within healthcare. This nuanced approach, thoughtfully embedded in legal and ethical frameworks, equips healthcare professionals to meet their duty of candour with confidence and compassion, turning the most challenging conversations into moments of profound connection and healing.

Legal and Professional Considerations

In the complex landscape of healthcare, where human vulnerability intertwines with technical precision, navigating the legal and professional considerations of candour requires a delicate and informed balance. Practising openness after an adverse event involves more than simply telling the truth; it requires a nuanced approach that honours both the dignity of patients and families and the legitimate protective frameworks that clinicians and organisations rely on. Central to this balancing act is the role of apology, a powerful, humanising gesture that can catalyse healing and restore trust, yet one that must be carefully crafted to avoid unintended legal ramifications.

At its core, apology serves as a bridge connecting the emotional experience of harm with the ethical responsibility of healthcare professionals. It acknowledges suffering without negating the serious responsibility borne by caregivers. Recognising when to apologise is pivotal, demanding situational awareness and emotional intelligence. It is neither an optional courtesy nor an automatic confession of fault; rather, it is a timely expression of empathy and regret for the impact of an incident on a patient's well-being. The moment to offer an apology is ideally as soon as the situation is sufficiently understood to communicate honestly, while still respecting the internal investigation process to avoid conjecture or premature conclusions. This timing represents a crossroads where transparency and caution must coalesce.

What an apology includes is equally consequential. Patients and families seek recognition of their distress and a sincere explanation of what happened, expressed in unambiguous language free from jargon or defensive distancing. However, professional boundaries must be strictly maintained to ensure that acknowledgement of harm does not become an admission of legal liability. Phrases such as "I am sorry for what you have experienced" or "We regret that this happened" convey compassion without direct blame. This careful framing allows clinicians to affirm their commitment to patient welfare and accountability without inadvertently exposing themselves or their organisations to litigation risks. Crafting such messages is a skilled art, one informed by legal counsel yet delivered with human warmth and humility.

The legal dimension of the duty of candour is multifaceted and varies across jurisdictions, yet common threads run through all contexts. The principle that honesty fosters patient safety and trust is widely endorsed, but this principle must be reconciled against the distinct legal environments where disclosures can be used in malpractice proceedings. Some healthcare systems provide statutory protection for certain disclosures or apologies, recognising that this openness ultimately reduces harm and promotes learning. Elsewhere, apologetic statements may be admissible as evidence, potentially complicating the clinician's position. This reality necessitates tailored institutional policies and training that help staff navigate these waters, ensuring that candour does not inadvertently increase vulnerability. The guidance rendered by legal teams is essential but cannot supplant the clinician's role as a compassionate communicator; instead, it equips professionals with the frameworks and phrases needed to honour both ethical obligations and legal prudence.

Maintaining professional boundaries during disclosure conversations is critical to preserving trust without compromising legal or organisational standing. While it is tempting after a distressing event to convey overt remorse or to engage in defensive explanations, doing so may destabilise these boundaries. Professionals must hold firm to their roles as empathetic informants rather than advocates or negotiators, recognising that their primary duty is patient well-being and truthful communication rather than apportioning blame. This distinction is especially salient in multi-disciplinary healthcare organisations where responsibility may be diffuse. Clear internal roles and support systems enable individuals to maintain this balance, ensuring that candour is practised consistently and ethically.

Moreover, risk management and candour are not adversarial but can, in fact, be complementary when approached with maturity and foresight. Concealing adverse events or deflecting accountability may offer ephemeral protections but ultimately erode trust and leave systemic issues unaddressed. Transparency, when skilfully managed within legal guardrails, promotes a culture of safety where errors are treated as opportunities for learning rather than occasions for concealment. This culture not only benefits patients through improved care quality but also protects healthcare professionals from the corrosive stress of secrecy. Leaders who champion this balanced approach enable clinicians to disclose with confidence, knowing that their honesty will be supported and contextualised appropriately.

Thus, the practice of apology within the duty of candour transcends a simplistic formula of words. It is a profound intersection where the human need for acknowledgment meets the professional imperative for prudence. Achieving this balance requires ongoing education, reflective practice, and institutional commitment to policies that integrate legal guidance with ethical clarity. When healthcare professionals are equipped to express genuine remorse without exposing themselves to undue risk, they contribute to a healthcare environment where mistakes become catalysts for healing and improvement, rather than sources of fear and mistrust. This equilibrium fosters resilience among clinicians and restores confidence among patients, embodying the true spirit of duty of candour.

Documentation, Reporting and Record-Keeping

Principles of Effective Documentation

The task of documentation in the context of duty of candour is one of profound responsibility and subtle nuance, demanding an unwavering commitment to clarity, accuracy, and comprehensiveness. At the heart of effective documentation lies the principle that what is recorded serves as a permanent, unaltered narrative of events, a truthful chronology that not only supports accountability but also becomes a critical tool for reflection, learning, and improvement. To document within this framework is to capture the essence of what transpired with meticulous detail, avoiding assumptions and subjective interpretations, while ensuring that the record is accessible, legible, and preserved according to established standards. The very act of documenting is intertwined with the ethical obligation to be transparent and truthful, particularly in the wake of adverse events where clarity can ease the distress of patients, families, and colleagues alike, while also guarding against misinformation and misunderstanding.

Documentation must begin with a clear, factual account of the incident as soon as possible after it occurs. Timeliness in recording is essential; memories fade, perceptions become clouded with time, and the opportunity to provide an accurate representation diminishes. Capturing details at the outset safeguards the integrity of the account and demonstrates a conscientious approach to professional responsibility. This initial record should focus on objective information: what happened, where and when it occurred, who was involved, and the circumstances surrounding the event. The narrative should describe actions taken immediately after the event, including any clinical interventions or communications initiated. It is vital to differentiate between observed facts and any personal reflections or opinions, which should be avoided or clearly identified and appropriately contextualised. Using language that is precise and unambiguous is critical, as documentation is relied upon not only internally but may also form the basis of communication with external agencies, regulators, and, if necessary, legal proceedings.

What exactly to record involves a balance between comprehensiveness and relevance. The documentation should include the initial identification of the incident, how and by whom it was recognised, as well as any early assessments made of the potential harm or risk. Details of the patient's response and condition changes at the time should be documented with exact times, clinical signs, symptoms, and any immediate diagnostic or therapeutic actions. This creates a robust timeline and contextual understanding necessary for any future investigation or review. Equally, the communication that follows an incident, particularly relating to explanations or apologies made to patients and families, must be carefully recorded. Here, the specific words used, the responses received, and any follow-up plans agreed upon should be noted comprehensively, as these records demonstrate the healthcare professional's adherence to the duty of candour and serve as evidence of their empathetic engagement.

Beyond the event itself and subsequent communication, good documentation integrates reflections on the incident's impact on care plans and any changes instituted to prevent recurrence. This might include noting referrals for support services for the patient or family, adjustments in treatment protocols, and involvement of multidisciplinary teams or patient safety committees. Each of these segments contributes to a fuller picture of how the incident was managed holistically. Furthermore, noting any discussions with colleagues or supervisors provides transparency regarding collaborative decision-making processes. Such records should detail who was consulted, the nature of their input, and the outcomes of these discussions. This approach not only supports internal accountability but fosters a culture of openness, showing that adverse events are collectively owned and addressed rather than concealed or minimised.

The format of the documentation itself demands thoughtful attention. Many organisations employ specific templates or digital platforms designed to facilitate comprehensive recording. These tools often mandate inclusion of critical elements, such as incident descriptions, contributing factors, immediate responses, communication logs, and follow-up actions, thereby standardising the quality and completeness of reports. Adhering to prescribed formats ensures consistency and legal compliance, making it easier for all stakeholders to locate and interpret key information efficiently. It also aids in reducing individual bias by guiding reporters to include all necessary data points rather than relying on freeform narrative that may omit essential details. For clinicians, familiarity with these templates before incidents occur improves readiness and confidence, allowing documentation to be completed rapidly and thoroughly without added stress or uncertainty.

Record retention policies form a crucial pillar supporting the integrity and utility of documentation. Healthcare organisations must maintain records for periods dictated by regulatory frameworks and internal governance, which often extend for several years beyond the event. Proper secure storage, whether in locked physical files or encrypted digital systems, preserves confidentiality and protects sensitive information from unauthorised access or potential loss. Maintaining accessibility within these constraints ensures that records remain available for audits, investigations, and, if necessary, disclosure to patients or legal representatives. Clarity around retention timelines also informs the process of transferring care or closing cases, helping professionals understand when documents may be formally archived or destroyed according to policy without compromising ongoing transparency.

Maintaining confidentiality throughout the documentation process is non-negotiable, given the sensitive nature of the information and the rights of patients and families. Records must be kept within secure systems that limit access to authorised personnel only, and when sharing is necessary, such as with regulators or external consultants, it should be governed by strict protocols and consent where applicable. Documentation should avoid extraneous personal identifiers beyond those relevant to the care context, and clinical notes should be recorded in a way that respects patient dignity and privacy. This ethical obligation supports not only legal compliance but also the preservation of trust, reinforcing that openness about adverse events does not translate into careless risk of exposure or harm to those involved.

The imperative for objectivity extends to the language used in documentation. Avoidance of emotive or judgmental wording cannot be overstressed. Descriptions such as "the patient was non-compliant" or "the team failed" should be replaced with neutral observations like "the patient declined the proposed treatment" or "a delay occurred between identification and intervention." This discipline protects healthcare professionals from unintended admissions of liability while ensuring the focus remains on facts and system improvements rather than individual blame. Similarly, the use of abbreviations and jargon should be limited and only employed when universally understood within the organisation, to avoid confusion or misinterpretation during handovers or reviews.

Documentation also plays a pivotal role in patient and family engagement. Transparent records form the foundation for discussions about what occurred, bolstering honesty and helping to rebuild trust damaged by the incident. When well-maintained records exist, healthcare professionals are better equipped to provide accurate information, avoid inconsistencies, and demonstrate that the situation was handled with care and responsibility. Moreover, documentation supports the principle of providing families with continuous updates and the opportunity to ask questions, further embedding candour into the culture of care. This active sharing of information, anchored in thorough records, challenges the old paradigm of secrecy and denial, pushing healthcare systems toward accountability and healing.

In addition to individual responsibility, documentation under the duty of candour must reflect organisational policies and legal standards, which often frame the content and detail required. Regulatory bodies across jurisdictions impose guidelines compelling healthcare providers to record incidents fully and accurately, as part of broader patient safety and quality assurance mandates. Failure to document appropriately can have far-reaching consequences, not only risk professional censure but also undermining the integrity of investigations and the possibility of learning from mistakes. Thus, documentation is more than an administrative exercise; it is a critical safety mechanism and a form of professional respect toward those served by the healthcare system.

The integration of documentation within a broader reporting and analysis framework further amplifies its value. Incident reports derived from documentation feed into quality improvement initiatives, root cause analyses, and policy revisions, turning individual adverse events into opportunities for systemic enhancement. By ensuring that records are precise and detailed, healthcare teams provide the raw material necessary for these processes to be meaningful and effective. This linkage between documentation and continuous improvement highlights the far-reaching impact of careful recording not only on immediate patient care but on the future reliability and safety of the entire healthcare delivery environment.

When considering documentation formats, it is essential to embrace technological advancements while preserving core principles of security and accuracy. Electronic health records (EHRs) offer tremendous advantages in real-time data entry, standardisation, and accessibility, but they also introduce challenges related to data integrity, user interface design, and potential overreliance on templates that might obscure individualised information. Professionals must be trained not only in system use but also in maintaining the narrative's nuance within electronic constraints, ensuring that documentation remains a true reflection of complex human events rather than sterile checkboxes. Additionally, regular audits of electronic records can help identify gaps, inconsistencies, or tendencies toward cursory entries, enabling continuous refinement of documentation practices.

Documentation under duty of candour is not a static task but an evolving practice that requires periodic reassessment. Organisations should foster an environment where clinicians are supported and educated on effective recording, recognising that good documentation is part of compassionate care and professional excellence. Feedback loops, reflective sessions, and peer reviews can enhance skills, reduce anxiety around reporting adverse events, and embed documentation as a valued component of clinical routine. This cultural reinforcement helps dismantle fears that documentation leads only to blame, reshaping it as a proactive instrument for protection, learning, and communication.

In conclusion, the principles of effective documentation within the duty of candour encompass a commitment to clear, accurate, timely, and comprehensive recording of adverse events, communications, and subsequent actions. Emphasising objective language, confidentiality, and compliance with policies ensures that documentation not only honours ethical obligations but also strengthens trust with patients and families. By embracing standardised formats, secure record retention, and the integration of technological tools, healthcare professionals safeguard the utility and integrity of their records. Beyond legal necessity, documentation is a foundational act of honesty and professionalism that helps transform difficult moments into learning opportunities and ultimately drives safer, more transparent care for all.

Reporting Protocols and Procedures

In the intricate tapestry of healthcare environments, where the stakes hinge on human life and well-being, the act of reporting adverse events treads a delicate yet fundamental path, one that demands precision, timeliness, and unwavering adherence to established protocols. Reporting protocols and procedures stand as the backbone of the duty of candour, forming a structured response that ensures transparency while safeguarding both patients and healthcare professionals. Clear, factual, and timely documentation acts not merely as a bureaucratic necessity but as a pivotal instrument in fostering trust, facilitating learning, and meeting the rigorous demands of legal and ethical frameworks. Within this complex landscape, understanding the internal and external requirements of incident reporting is essential for healthcare providers who must navigate multiple layers of responsibility.

Central to internal reporting protocols is the principle that documentation must be immediate and accurate. From the moment an adverse event or error occurs, healthcare professionals are expected to record the details with utmost clarity, avoiding assumptions, interpretations, or emotional language that can cloud the objective narrative. The initial report typically forms the first piece of the investigative puzzle and thus must capture the essential facts: what happened, when, where, who was involved, and the immediate consequences. This first-level documentation is often entered into risk management or incident reporting systems tailored to the institution's standards, providing a secure repository that enables systematic tracking, follow-up, and analysis. Such internal mechanisms are designed to promote consistency and ease of access, ensuring that all incidents, regardless of severity, receive appropriate attention and escalation according to predefined triage thresholds.

Within the organisational hierarchy, these protocols extend beyond mere data entry, requiring multidisciplinary involvement to contextualise the event and begin preliminary assessment. Management teams rely heavily on prompt reports to allocate resources efficiently and initiate preliminary risk assessments or initial remedial actions. Simultaneously, healthcare professionals maintain the duty to record their observations, decisions, and communications transparently, preserving a detailed chronology that can be revisited as investigations unfold. Confidentiality in documentation is stringently maintained; personnel must balance openness with discretion, ensuring that sensitive information is shared only on a need-to-know basis within the institution, thereby preserving patient privacy and professional trust.

Externally, reporting obligations invoke additional layers of complexity. Healthcare organisations operate within a regulatory ecosystem that may mandate the escalation of certain adverse events to external bodies such as national patient safety authorities, healthcare regulators, or public health agencies. These bodies often require formal incident reports, which, while similar in nature to internal documentation, may have distinct formats, scopes, and submission timelines. For example, serious adverse events or 'never events' designated as occurrences that should never happen if appropriate care standards are met are subject to almost immediate external notification to facilitate oversight, public accountability, and system -wide learning. Compliance with these external reporting demands not only fulfils legal obligations but also signals a commitment to transparency and patient safety on a broader scale. Failure to comply can carry significant consequences, including reputational damage, financial penalties, or even regulatory sanctions.

The preparation of external reports demands scrupulous attention to accuracy and completeness, with narratives carefully constructed to reflect an impartial recounting of events supported by documented evidence. Often, these submissions are facilitated through standardised forms that incorporate critical categories such as patient demographics, incident description, contributory factors, and outcome severity. Some regulatory frameworks further require organisations to submit action plans or evidence of remedial measures alongside incident reports, illustrating a proactive approach to risk mitigation. Interfacing with external regulators necessitates a respectful collaboration, acknowledging their role not as punitive enforcers but as partners in advancing healthcare safety. Thus, the dual nature of reporting internally for organisational learning and externally for regulatory compliance must be harmonised within a cohesive strategy.

Integral to both internal and external reporting procedures are organisational policies that delineate record retention timelines and confidentiality safeguards. Healthcare institutions often establish retention periods mirroring statutory requirements to ensure that documentation remains available for future audits, legal proceedings, or retrospective analyses. These policies address storage formats ranging from secure physical archives to encrypted digital repositories that protect against unauthorised access while enabling timely retrieval. Safeguarding patient-identifiable data adheres to stringent privacy laws that mandate anonymisation or controlled access to prevent breaches. Equally, healthcare professionals contributing to the documentation process are typically afforded safeguards regarding the use of their records, with mechanisms in place to prevent persecution or undue disciplinary action when reporting incidents in good faith.

The confidentiality surrounding reports is paramount not only for patient privacy but also for fostering a culture in which healthcare workers feel psychologically safe disclosing errors. Mechanisms such as anonymised reporting channels, de-identified data submission, and protected communication spaces help mitigate fear of blame and encourage candour. This cultural dimension complements procedural rigour, as the efficacy of reporting systems depends equally on how they are perceived by frontline staff. Trust in the reporting framework encourages compliance and enriches the quality of information, which in turn catalyses effective investigations and meaningful improvements in patient safety.

Importantly, reporting protocols are neither static nor isolated; they evolve in response to emerging evidence, technological advances, and legislative changes. Institutions often review and update their procedures to incorporate best practices, such as integrating real-time electronic health record systems with incident reporting tools, enabling seamless data capture and reducing administrative burden. Training programs are critical components that bolster healthcare professionals' familiarity with reporting requirements and emphasise the importance of promptness, completeness, and accuracy. Simulation exercises and scenario-based learning help embed procedural knowledge, ensuring that in moments of high stress, staff are equipped to fulfil their duties consistently.

Lastly, the interplay between reporting and communication with patients and families cannot be overstated. Documentation of adverse events serves as a foundational resource for openness initiatives that include timely disclosure and apology. Clear records provide the factual basis for compassionate conversations, enabling healthcare professionals to convey honesty without speculation. In this way, reporting protocols contribute not only to organisational accountability but also to repairing and maintaining the therapeutic alliance that has been damaged by harm.

In conclusion, mastering the intricate web of internal and external reporting protocols and procedures is essential for healthcare professionals committed to practising the duty of candour. The rigorous recording, retention, and confidentiality of incident reports embody healthcare organisations' commitment to transparency, learning, and continuous improvement. By faithfully adhering to these frameworks, professionals not only comply with legal and ethical mandates but also nurture trust both within their teams and with the patients they serve, transforming moments of misfortune into catalysts for safer, more compassionate care.

Maintaining Confidentiality and Security

In the demanding sphere of healthcare, maintaining confidentiality and security of patient information is not merely a procedural obligation but an ethical imperative that underpins every aspect of care delivery and professional communication. The duty of candour, which calls for openness and honesty when things go wrong, must always be balanced with a steadfast commitment to protecting sensitive patient data. The responsibility healthcare professionals bear extends beyond the immediate clinical context to encompass every narrative, report, and interaction involving patient information. This safeguarding is critical because the ramifications of compromised confidentiality can be profound, ranging from loss of trust and potential harm to patients and families to serious legal consequences for individuals and organisations alike. Understanding the landscape of confidentiality within the duty of candour framework requires an appreciation of the intricate interplay among transparency, privacy, and professional accountability.

At the initial stage, when an adverse event occurs, clinicians and other healthcare providers often face the dual challenges of documenting the incident comprehensively and communicating clearly with the affected patient or family. Meticulous documentation is vital, yet it must be carried out with unwavering attention to confidentiality. Every entry must reflect a clear, factual recounting of what transpired, avoiding subjective assumptions or conjecture. This accuracy is essential not only for clarity and future reference but also for safeguarding the patient's medical narrative from distortion or unauthorised disclosure. The documentation captures delicate personal data and clinical details that, if mishandled, could expose patients to social stigma, psychological distress, or even discrimination. Thus, healthcare professionals must be trained to balance detail with discretion, ensuring that records contain sufficient information for investigation and learning without revealing unnecessary personal identifiers beyond those authorised by policies or regulations.

Security of these records is equally paramount. With the pervasive adoption of digital health records, safeguarding patient information now involves navigating complex cyber environments, where the threat of hacking, accidental breaches, or unauthorised access looms large. Practising the duty of candour requires institutions to deploy robust technological defences, including encryption, access controls, and secure authentication processes, to protect the integrity of electronic records. Physical safeguards are no less important in environments where paper records still exist; secure filing systems with restricted access, surveillance, and designated confidentiality zones are essential measures. Professionals must also be vigilant with oral communication, recognising that dialogue about incidents or patient information should never occur in public or unsecured spaces, and that conversations must remain confidential within the circle of care.

Confidentiality is not only a point of clinical ethics but also a cornerstone of legal compliance. Healthcare organisations operate within a regulatory framework designed to enforce stringent protections for patient data. Legislation such as the Health Insurance Portability and Accountability Act (HIPAA) in the United States, the General Data Protection Regulation (GDPR) in Europe, and other jurisdictional standards impose strict conditions on how information may be collected, used, shared, and stored. These laws require that pertinent reports following adverse events are handled under strict confidentiality protocols and reveal only what is necessary for legal or quality assurance purposes. Moreover, compliance extends beyond technical adherence; it encompasses cultivating an institutional culture in which privacy is respected, and every member of the healthcare team understands their role in safeguarding data. This culture promotes vigilance and accountability, discouraging informal sharing or careless handling of information that might inadvertently breach confidentiality.

In practical terms, report formats following duty of candour incidents must be carefully designed to align with confidentiality requirements. Templates should guide healthcare professionals to focus on factual, clinical descriptions and omit extraneous personal data unless directly relevant. These templates also aid in standardising the documentation process, reducing variability that might lead to incomplete or potentially revealing content. Simultaneously, organisations must maintain clear, accessible policies that guide record retention, define the duration and conditions under which sensitive information is stored, and ensure archives are secure against tampering or loss. Retention policies must also consider legal mandates that prescribe minimum and maximum periods for retaining patient data, balancing the need for long-term availability in the event of litigation or audits against the risks inherent in prolonged data retention.

The custodial role of healthcare managers and designated privacy officers is critical to the oversight of confidentiality practices. They are responsible for implementing regular training programs that emphasise the nuances of the duty of candour and confidentiality, keeping staff abreast of evolving legal requirements and best-practice standards. Beyond training, these leaders must establish audit mechanisms and feedback loops to monitor compliance, identify vulnerabilities, and address breaches swiftly and transparently. This oversight fosters trust among clinical teams that confidentiality is taken seriously and encourages the prompt reporting of any lapses without fear of retribution, which itself is essential for continuous improvement and learning from incidents.

Communicating with patients and families during disclosure processes inherently involves handling highly sensitive information. The dialogue must preserve individuals' dignity and privacy, providing them with the information necessary to understand what happened while protecting them from unnecessary exposure or embarrassment. This calls for a considered approach to verbal and written communication, ensuring that shared details are relevant and respectful. Confidentiality extends to the management of patients' emotional responses and personal narratives; healthcare professionals must ensure private environments for discussions and obtain consent before involving third parties or external advisors. Throughout this process, transparency and confidentiality are not opposing forces but rather coexisting principles that require careful navigation and skilful balance.

Healthcare professionals must also guard against the inadvertent spread of information through modern communication channels such as social media, email, and informal chats among colleagues. Social media's pervasive reach demands caution, as what may begin as a seemingly innocuous comment or post can escalate into a public breach, eroding patient trust and exposing institutions to reputational and legal damage. Thus, the duty of candour must be embedded within wider professional conduct standards, reminding all healthcare workers that maintaining confidentiality is integral to their professional identity and public credibility.

When breaches do occur, a transparent yet confidential response is critical. Organisations must have clear protocols for investigating breaches, managing harm, and mitigating risks of further exposure. Responses should be handled with sensitivity to affected patients, with disclosures made in accordance with legal advice and ethical standards to restore trust, mend relationships, and demonstrate organisational accountability. Learning from breaches is a vital component of an evolving duty of candour framework, reinforcing the importance of continuous education and system improvements to prevent recurrence.

In conclusion, protecting patient information within the duty of candour practice stands as a fundamental pillar supporting both the ethical and practical dimensions of healthcare transparency. It requires a vigilant, informed approach that integrates secure documentation practices, compliance with legal standards, robust institutional policies, and a culture of trust deeply embedded in every level of the healthcare system. By upholding confidentiality and security alongside candour, healthcare professionals advance not only the immediate interests of patient safety and dignity but also the broader goals of organisational integrity, public confidence, and the transformative potential of openness in healthcare. The challenge is ongoing, demanding continuous reflection, adaptation, and a heartfelt commitment to respecting the sacred trust patients place in their caregivers every time they share their stories, vulnerabilities, and lives.

Working with Regulators and Legal Teams

Understanding Regulatory Processes

When an adverse event occurs in healthcare, the involvement of regulatory bodies and external oversight is an inevitable part of the journey towards resolution and improvement. For many clinicians and managers, the prospect of interacting with regulators or investigators can provoke anxiety or uncertainty, particularly when the processes and expectations are not fully understood. Yet, viewing these interactions through a lens of preparedness and partnership rather than confrontation opens the door to constructive engagement and, ultimately, better outcomes for patients and organisations alike.

At its essence, regulatory oversight in healthcare serves a dual purpose: protecting the public by ensuring safe, ethical care and fostering an environment of accountability and continuous learning within healthcare systems. Regulators are charged with examining adverse events and clinical incidents not as punitive arbiters, but as guardians of patient safety standards and professional integrity. This fundamental perspective can help healthcare professionals, from frontline clinicians to senior managers, appreciate the role these external bodies play as part of a broader safety net, rather than as adversarial forces.

When a report or complaint reaches a regulatory authority, the first step you can expect is a formal review process designed to assess the nature and scope of the incident. This may involve detailed requests for documentation, timelines, and narratives from individuals involved. Understanding this preparatory phase is crucial, as it sets the tone for subsequent investigations or hearings. Regulators seek clear, accurate information that reflects diligent internal review and candour in disclosure. Healthcare professionals should therefore gather records methodically and support answers with factual evidence whenever possible, avoiding speculation or assumptions. Transparent and organised communication at this stage demonstrates respect for the regulator's oversight role and can prevent unnecessary prolonging of the inquiry.

The process that follows often includes visits or interviews conducted by inspectors, investigators, or panels appointed by the regulatory agency. These interactions are not adversarial examinations but structured conversations to clarify facts, understand context, and identify system deficiencies. Clinicians and managers have the right to be accompanied by a support person, legal advisor, or professional representative during these meetings, ensuring that their perspective is fairly presented and protected. Being well-prepared for this engagement means reviewing relevant case details, anticipating potential questions, and rehearsing clear, calm explanations that acknowledge what is known while openly admitting uncertainties or errors. The aim is to foster mutual trust between the regulated party and the regulator through honesty and professionalism.

While regulatory scrutiny naturally raises concerns about possible disciplinary actions or legal ramifications, it is vital to distinguish the investigative purpose from any eventual enforcement decisions Regulatory bodies may make recommendations, require remedial actions, or escalate matters to licensing boards, but the initial phases predominantly focus on understanding the incident's root causes and identifying opportunities for system-wide improvements. Healthcare professionals should approach the process with a constructive mindset, viewing the oversight as a chance to contribute toward safer practices, rather than exclusively a defensively motivated exercise. This reframing supports both personal resilience and organisational culture shifts toward openness.

Communication with regulators requires a delicate balance between openness and legal awareness. It is common to worry that full transparency might inadvertently expose professionals or organisations to increased liability. However, research and practical experience reveal that openness and sincerity often enhance credibility and reduce mistrust, which can sometimes mitigate harsher repercussions. Nevertheless, it remains essential for healthcare workers to understand their rights, including the right to seek legal counsel prior to or during regulatory interactions, the right to access investigative findings, and the right to appeal or respond to agency decisions. Being informed about these rights empowers individuals to participate fully and assertively in the regulatory processes while safeguarding their interests.

Preparation is not limited to individuals alone; healthcare managers and organisational leaders play a pivotal role in equipping their teams for productive eyes-on oversight. Establishing clear internal protocols for handling regulatory inquiries, training staff in effective communication and documentation, and fostering a non-punitive culture that values learning over blame all contribute to smoother engagements. When clinicians and managers see regulatory involvement as part of a broader cycle that includes incident reporting, patient disclosure, internal investigation, and external review, it normalises the process as one linked to growth rather than fear.

Frequently, healthcare organisations encounter different types of regulators, each with distinct responsibilities and approaches, thus making general familiarity important. For example, professional licensing bodies tend to focus on individual conduct and competence, often reviewing whether practitioners meet accepted standards. On the other hand, health system oversight agencies might examine organisational policies, systemic failures, and overall patient safety practices. Additionally, statutory bodies tasked with investigating serious incidents might prioritise fact-finding to protect the public and prevent future harm. Knowing which entity is involved and their remit aids in targeting the response appropriately and understanding what information is likely to be requested or reviewed.

During regulatory reviews, one should expect a degree of scrutiny that extends beyond the individual incident. Investigators commonly explore the broader context of staffing levels, training adequacy, equipment functionality, communication systems, and leadership support to identify latent conditions that contributed to the event. Consequently, factual accuracy in reporting is critical, but so is the awareness that the findings may lead to recommendations or requirements for systemic changes. This is often the regulatory process's greatest value: highlighting the interconnected factors that affect patient safety and prompting improvements that benefit future care.

Engagement with legal advisors during regulatory processes is another important consideration for healthcare professionals. Legal counsel can clarify the implications of disclosure, help navigate complex procedural requirements, and advise on the boundaries of privileged communication. For instance, some regulatory interviews and reports may be protected from being interpreted as admissions of liability, but such protections can vary by jurisdiction and case specifics. Understanding these nuances can prevent missteps that complicate defences or organisational reputations. In addition, proactive collaboration between legal teams and clinical leaders ensures that candour is practised safely, honouring both ethical imperatives and risk management principles.

Experienced regulators often emphasise that timely cooperation strengthens relationships and expedites resolution. Delays in responding to enquiries or withholding information can raise suspicion and prolong investigations. Healthcare providers should therefore adopt a policy of promptness combined with accuracy, communicating realistic timelines for collating information and clearly indicating when further details will be available. When difficulties arise, such as lost records or unclear accounts, transparency about these issues, rather than concealment, is crucial for maintaining trust. Demonstrating openness from the outset not only assists the regulatory body but also reflects the ethos central to the Duty of Candour.

While regulators primarily serve to protect patients and ensure quality, they also recognise the emotional toll that investigations impose on healthcare professionals. Sensitivity in communication, empathy for the professionals involved, and provision of support resources can all be part of regulatory practice. Knowing this helps clinicians and managers to engage without feeling unduly threatened or isolated. Organisations can reinforce this approach by fostering peer support structures and offering mental well-being interventions for staff caught up in such reviews, thereby sustaining a healthy workforce capable of continuous learning.

An additional dimension of the regulatory process involves the interface between external reviews and internal organisational governance. Many healthcare providers must balance the demands of regulatory compliance with their own risk management, clinical governance, and quality improvement frameworks. Regulators typically encourage integration of their findings into ongoing improvement initiatives rather than treating their input as a standalone event. This means leadership must be prepared not only to facilitate transparency with external bodies but also to translate feedback into measurable action plans, monitor implementation, and close the feedback loop with their teams. Such integration enhances the perceived value of regulatory engagement and strengthens an organisation's safety culture.

Moreover, healthcare professionals should anticipate that regulatory reviews may culminate in formal reports, recommendations, or notices. These documents often provide a detailed synthesis of the investigation's findings, highlight both strengths and weaknesses, and suggest corrective measures ranging from additional training and policy changes to monitoring and, in rare cases, disciplinary sanctions. Reading and understanding these reports thoroughly is essential to ensure compliance and to identify any opportunities for clarification or appeal. Involving multidisciplinary teams in reviewing outcomes promotes a shared understanding and collective ownership of improvement efforts driven by regulatory input.

Importantly, the duty to disclose adverse events to patients and families intersects significantly with regulatory processes. Transparency with those affected aligns with both ethical obligations and regulatory expectations. Regulators value evidence that healthcare providers have responsibly informed patients and offered appropriate apologies and support before or during investigations. Demonstrating this responsible candour not only builds external trust but also protects the provider from additional scrutiny or criticism for secrecy or evasiveness. It reinforces the idea that open dialogue, both internally and with patients, is an anchor that sustains integrity through challenging times.

In summary, the regulatory oversight experience, though often perceived as intimidating, can be reframed as an essential pillar of accountable, high-quality healthcare. Understanding what regulators expect, how to communicate effectively with them, and how to use the process as an opportunity for learning and improvement delivers significant benefits for clinicians, managers, and healthcare organisations alike. Preparing thoughtfully for regulatory interactions while honouring professional responsibilities and rights nurtures confidence during reviews. It empowers stakeholders to uphold the duty of candour with integrity, transforming difficult moments into catalysts for safer, more transparent care for all patients.

Preparing for Legal Inquiries

Facing legal inquiries in the aftermath of an adverse event can be one of the most daunting experiences for healthcare professionals and managers alike. The atmosphere is often charged with anxiety, uncertainty, and a profound sense of responsibility that weighs heavily on those involved. However, preparation is the cornerstone that transforms this intimidating process into a manageable, even empowering, opportunity to demonstrate integrity and commitment to patient safety. When clinicians and healthcare managers understand how to document comprehensively and present their cases effectively, they can navigate legal inquiries with confidence and clarity, mitigating potential harm to their professional reputations while upholding the principles of candour.

The first step in preparing for any legal inquiry is to adopt a mindset that embraces transparency without sacrificing prudence. It is essential to remember that documenting an incident meticulously is not merely a clerical task but a vital part of the accountability mechanism within healthcare. Every note, every report, every communication can become a piece of evidence in an investigation. Thus, when you write, you are, in essence, creating a narrative that reflects your professional conduct and decision-making in real time. This narrative must be accurate, objective, and unambiguous. Avoid speculation, assumptions, or emotional language; instead, focus on facts. Record what happened, when it happened, who was involved, what actions you took, and any conversations or instructions given. This disciplined approach to documentation helps to build a robust foundation of credibility that will support you throughout an inquiry.

Recognising the significance of consistency in all documentation cannot be overstated. Discrepancies in accounts, however minor they may seem, can cast shadows of doubt and invite scrutiny. Therefore, clinicians and managers should regularly review their records to ensure that information is consistent across documents and communication channels. If discrepancies arise for valid reasons, such as new information coming to light, it is crucial to document the updates clearly and explain the context. This transparent approach fosters trust with investigators and legal advisors, who are trained to spot inconsistencies and are likely to probe deeply when the narrative does not cohere.

Equally important is understanding the regulatory environment and legal frameworks that govern duty of candour practices in your jurisdiction. While the ethical imperative to disclose harm honestly is universal, the legal implications and procedural requirements can vary widely across healthcare systems and local laws. Engaging proactively with your institution's legal department and compliance officers can illuminate these nuances. They can brief you on your rights and responsibilities, help interpret relevant legislation, and advise on how to structure your disclosures and responses to inquiries in ways that are compliant yet forthright. This collaboration is vital because it balances the need for openness with prudent legal risk management, reducing anxiety by ensuring you are not navigating these complex waters alone.

Effective preparation also involves anticipating the kinds of questions or challenges that may arise during a legal review. Regulators and legal representatives often focus on establishing timelines, determining the adequacy of care provided, evaluating communication between staff and patients, and assessing whether organisational policies were followed. Preparing for these inquiries requires you to revisit the entire case thoroughly, understand the clinical decisions made, and be ready to explain your rationale clearly and calmly. Role-playing or mock interviews facilitated by legal or compliance teams can be invaluable in this regard, helping you to articulate your responses with confidence and to remain composed under pressure.

When it comes to interactions with regulators or legal investigators, communication is an art that blends honesty with strategic thinking. It is crucial to maintain a tone of respect and cooperation, as antagonism can alienate those responsible for impartial review and potentially escalate tensions. At the same time, it is wise to avoid volunteering excessive information that is not explicitly requested or that could inadvertently jeopardise your position. Consulting with legal advisors beforehand to develop key messages ensures that your responses are precise, legally sound, and consistent. You should also clarify if you have the right to have a representative present during interviews or meetings, as this can provide not only emotional support but also practical assistance in interpreting questions and framing answers appropriately.

Document representation goes hand in hand with verbal communication. When documents are requested as part of a legal inquiry, the presentation and organisation of these materials should be meticulous. Provide clear, well-labelled copies with a summary or index highlighting relevant sections to guide reviewers efficiently through the evidence. This consideration demonstrates your professionalism and respect for the inquiry process. It can also influence perceptions positively by showing that you take the matter seriously and are committed to transparency.

Another critical component of preparing for legal inquiries is managing internal communications within your healthcare organisation. It is common for teams to feel apprehensive or defensive after an adverse event, which can lead to defensiveness or conflicting narratives. As a leader or clinician, you have a responsibility to foster a culture that encourages and supports honest dialogue. Encouraging staff to document their perspectives accurately and share concerns early can prevent surprises during external investigations. When everyone understands that the duty of candour is not about blame but about learning and improvement, teams become more cohesive and resilient, ultimately strengthening the organisation's legal and ethical position.

One must also be mindful of the potential emotional toll that legal inquiries can exact on individuals involved. The fear of litigation, loss of professional status, or reputational damage can cause stress and even ethical dilemmas about how much to disclose. Healthcare professionals should seek support from peers, mentors, or counselling services when needed to maintain psychological well-being. Staying grounded and focused on the core values of patient care and honesty helps sustain motivation and clarity during challenging legal processes.

It is vital to remember that legal inquiries aim, above all, to understand what happened and to prevent future harm. In this spirit, demonstrating a genuine commitment to learning, improvement, and patient safety can have a favourable impact on how your case is perceived. Proactively acknowledging errors where appropriate, outlining steps taken to mitigate risk, and participating constructively in investigations exemplify professional integrity. This approach does not diminish the seriousness of the inquiry; rather, it strengthens it by contributing to systemic solutions.

Timeliness is another critical factor in legal preparation. Delays or failures to provide requested information can cast doubt on an individual's or organisation's credibility and may have legal repercussions. Setting realistic but prompt timelines for collecting documentation, securing legal counsel, and preparing detailed responses is essential. Utilising project management tools or assigning clear roles within your team can facilitate this process, ensuring that no crucial aspect is overlooked under pressure.

The technical quality of documentation should not be ignored either. Handwritten notes should be legible and signed, and electronic records should be properly saved and backed up. Any alterations or corrections must follow accepted protocols and clearly show the original entries and the reasons for the changes. This attention to detail guards against accusations of tampering or misrepresentation, which can derail even well-intentioned efforts at transparency.

Furthermore, familiarity with the common procedural steps followed by regulatory and legal bodies helps reduce uncertainty. Knowing the phases of inquiry from initial notification, evidence gathering, interviews, to final reporting allows you to anticipate your involvement and prepare documentation accordingly. Some jurisdictions may have formal mechanisms for mediation or alternative dispute resolution, which can be less adversarial and provide earlier opportunities for resolution. Exploring these options with legal advice can be beneficial, especially when the goal is to restore trust with patients and families rather than merely to defend against liability.

For healthcare managers, an added layer of responsibility involves aligning institutional policies with the principles of duty of candour and ensuring staff are adequately trained in these areas. This preventative stance means fewer surprises during incidents and inquiries, as everyone understands the protocols for immediate response, documentation, and disclosure. When incidents occur, managers should ensure that team members have access to expert legal advice promptly and that communication with external bodies is coordinated and consistent.

It is also important to record and preserve any informal communications that relate to the incident or inquiry. Emails, phone call summaries, meeting minutes, and even text messages can become relevant pieces of evidence. Proper archiving processes must therefore be followed to maintain integrity and traceability. Conversely, be cautious about sharing opinions or speculations through informal channels, especially when they pertain to adverse events under investigation.

In the realm of legal inquiries, the interplay between the duty of candour and legal protections such as privilege or confidentiality can sometimes be complex. Knowing when to share information openly and when to seek legal guidance before disclosure is critical. For instance, certain jurisdictions provide safeguards for quality improvement discussions or root cause analyses that encourage frank reflection by protecting these communications from being used in litigation. Understanding how these protections operate and their limits can influence what information is documented and how it is presented during inquiries.

The narrative you construct in your documentation and verbal presentations ultimately must reflect a coherent story that acknowledges reality while contextualising decisions and actions taken in a complex clinical environment. Striving for this balance requires humility, self-awareness, and a commitment to ethical practice. It means admitting what is known, acknowledging uncertainties, and describing efforts made to address gaps or errors. This approach not only serves legal interests but, more importantly, preserves professional integrity and supports healing for all parties involved.

Preparing thoroughly for legal inquiries concerning the duty of candour is neither simple nor comforting, but it is indispensable. By embracing accuracy, consistency, collaboration with legal experts, professional communication, emotional resilience, and a learning mindset, healthcare professionals and managers can face these challenges with assurance. Ultimately, diligent preparation transforms potential vulnerability into demonstrated accountability and contributes to a culture of truth and safety that benefits patients, families, and care providers alike.

Collaboration and Communication Strategies

In the complex and often challenging landscape of healthcare, the moment an adverse event occurs and triggers scrutiny from regulators, investigators, or legal advisors is one where the interplay of professionalism and transparency becomes pivotal. When clinicians and healthcare managers find themselves navigating these waters, the dual imperative is clear: to maintain the highest standards of openness and candour without compromising the integrity or fairness of the process. This balancing act requires a deep understanding not only of what must be communicated but also of how and when to communicate it, as well as the ability to accurately discern rights and responsibilities within the frameworks of regulatory and legal oversight. Successfully managing this delicate equilibrium is foundational to upholding trust with all parties involved and ultimately advancing a culture of safety and learning within healthcare settings.

From the outset, preparation forms the bedrock of effective collaboration with external bodies. Healthcare professionals must recognise that participating in regulatory reviews or legal investigations is neither an adversarial confrontation nor a bureaucratic formality; rather, it is a critical opportunity to contribute to system-wide improvements while safeguarding patient interests and professional accountability. Preparation begins with a thorough and honest internal review of the incident in question, approaching the facts with clarity and emotional equanimity. This introspection involves gathering all relevant clinical records, timelines, witness statements, and any prior correspondences or reports connected to the event. Such meticulous documentation not only fortifies the responder's credibility but also ensures that communication remains clear, factual, and devoid of speculation or defensive distortion. The clarity gained through this reflective process also bolsters confidence, which is indispensable in interactions that might otherwise be intimidating or fraught with tension.

Communication strategies in this context must be rooted in respect, transparency, and active listening. When engaging with regulators or investigators, an open and patient-centred approach is vital, but it also requires a calibrated professionalism that guards against inadvertent misstatements. It is essential to recognise that the tone and substance of dialogue can significantly influence perceptions of sincerity and reliability. Healthcare professionals should approach conversations by calmly and clearly outlining their understanding of the incident, the clinical rationale underpinning decisions, and the steps already undertaken to address the harm or prevent recurrence. This not only demonstrates accountability but also respects the investigative process's intent to identify learning opportunities rather than apportion blame. Concomitantly, practitioners must be attuned to the questions posed, responding with transparency while refraining from conjecture. When answers are unknown or uncertain, it is both ethical and wise to acknowledge the limits of one's knowledge and affirm a commitment to follow up where appropriate.

The role of empathy in interactions with regulators and legal advisors is frequently underestimated but crucial in maintaining professionalism. While the encounters are inherently formal and procedural, the underlying human dimension, the impact of adverse events on patients, families, and healthcare teams, must remain foregrounded. Expressing a genuine commitment to patient safety and continuous improvement communicates that disclosure and collaboration are not mere obligations but part of a compassionate professional ethos. This stance can help transform a potentially adversarial interaction into a shared effort toward transparent accountability. Additionally, it influences the tone of the relationship beyond the immediate case, fostering trust and openness that can reverberate positively within the wider healthcare environment.

Understanding one's rights and responsibilities during these processes is equally essential. Healthcare professionals often face anxiety over potential legal repercussions or professional sanctions, which can act as barriers to candour and cooperation. Yet a well-grounded knowledge of the jurisdiction's legal protections and obligations greatly empowers clinicians and managers alike. The Duty of Candour, embedded in many healthcare systems, obliges openness and honest communication when harm occurs, while also providing frameworks to protect individuals who participate in disclosures and investigations in good faith. Therefore, clinicians should be familiar with institutional policies, statutory requirements, and relevant professional codes of conduct governing behavioural expectations during regulatory reviews. Understanding that transparency is not an act of self-incrimination, but a professional responsibility supported by legal safeguards, can reduce fears and encourage full engagement with investigatory processes.

Equally, professionals must be aware that regulators and legal advisors themselves are bound by codes that require impartiality, dignity, and respect for due process. Recognising this mutual responsibility for professionalism helps create constructive dialogues. It also reminds healthcare participants that, while their cooperation is expected, they are entitled to procedural fairness, including timely information about the process, clarification of the scope of the inquiries, and, where appropriate, access to support systems such as legal counsel or workplace advocates. This understanding transforms potentially opaque or intimidating processes into more navigable experiences characterised by transparency and respect.

When engaging with legal advisors, communication becomes even more nuanced. Legal professionals bring specialised expertise designed to protect the rights of both the healthcare provider and the patients or their families involved. Open communication with legal counsel is crucial, but it requires strategic clarity, given that legal advice often involves managing risk while maintaining obligations to truth and accountability. Clinicians and managers should approach these conversations with honesty and completeness, recognising that withholding or distorting information can severely compromise trust and outcomes. Conversely, legal advisors can help frame the candour process within the context of protective measures, guiding disclosures to remain truthful yet judicious, thereby minimising unnecessary legal vulnerability. This collaboration ensures that transparency is upheld without undermining the safety and sustainability of healthcare providers' professional positions.

The intersection of candour and legal processes also necessitates thoughtful timing in communication. While openness mandates timely disclosure and cooperation, rushing interactions without adequate preparation or reflection can jeopardise clarity and accuracy. Healthcare professionals should work with their organisations to establish clear protocols for when and how information is shared, ensuring that all communications to regulators or legal representatives follow a logical, coordinated pathway. This prevents conflicting messages, confusion, or inadvertent gaps in information that might hinder investigations or damage professional credibility. Hence, preparing and rehearsing key points, understanding the sequence of events, and practicing clear, empathetic wording become invaluable components of effective collaboration.

Another vital component of a communication strategy is the use of structured frameworks, or conversation guides, in dialogue with external bodies. Such tools assist in maintaining professionalism by providing consistent language that balances openness with discretion. They help avoid overly defensive or vague responses, thereby fostering credibility and trust. While flexibility must remain to respond authentically to specific inquiries, having a considered script or set of agreed-upon principles equips healthcare professionals to manage their emotional responses and maintain the professional composure necessary in high-stress environments. These frameworks can also ensure that communication covers critical areas such as acknowledgement of harm, description of immediate actions taken, and plans for systemic improvements, which are all key markers of credible candour.

Beyond individual interactions, successful collaboration with regulators and legal entities involves ongoing dialogue that emphasises learning and improvement. A purely transactional or event-driven mindset where communication ceases once a report is submitted or a review is completed misses the broader purpose of transparency. Continued open lines of communication can facilitate updates on remedial measures, feedback on system changes, and opportunities to participate in joint efforts for safety enhancement. Such a dynamic engenders stronger relationships, helping organisations and regulatory bodies work in partnership rather than opposition. This continuous engagement also demonstrates organisational maturity and commitment to candour as a systemic value, encouraging more thorough, fair, and constructive investigative processes.

Healthcare leaders play a crucial role in modelling and supporting these communication strategies. Their involvement ensures that clinicians do not feel isolated or vulnerable when external scrutiny arises. Leaders can foster environments were reaching out to legal or regulatory advisors is not stigmatised but embraced as a routine element of accountability and quality assurance. By providing practical support, training, and emotional resilience resources, managers help clinicians approach disclosures with greater confidence. Leaders also act as liaisons who can translate technical, legal or regulatory language into accessible terms for clinical teams, ensuring that professionals remain informed and empowered rather than confused or intimidated. In essence, leadership bridges the sometimes-disparate cultures of clinical care and regulatory compliance, creating synergy around transparency objectives.

In practice, several real-world examples highlight how professionalism and transparency can harmoniously coexist in these challenging circumstances. Consider a scenario where a nurse involved in a medication error is summoned for regulatory review. With appropriate preparation, guided by their manager and legal counsel, the nurse approaches the meeting openly, acknowledging the mistake while providing factual context and explaining systemic factors contributing to the incident. Rather than retreating into denial or self-blame, the nurse communicates a readiness to participate in corrective actions. Regulators respond by appreciating the candour and work collaboratively to recommend practical improvements. This cooperative approach not only preserves the nurse's professional dignity but also contributes to meaningful patient safety advancements.

Conversely, failing to maintain transparency or professionalism can have detrimental consequences, erode trust and complicate organisational culture. For example, evasion, incomplete disclosure, or defensive posturing in communications with legal or regulatory bodies can lead to prolonged investigations, loss of professional credibility, and damage to the institution's reputation. It may also foster mistrust from patients and families, who expect openness and truthfulness, and alienate healthcare teams, undermining morale and willingness to engage in future disclosure. Such outcomes serve as cautionary reminders of the necessity to embed professionalism and transparency as interdependent pillars during all phases of collaboration and communication.

Ultimately, collaboration and communication with regulators, investigators, and legal advisors represent more than procedural obligations; they are ethical imperatives that embody the very essence of the Duty of Candour. When healthcare professionals approach these interactions with preparedness, honesty, empathy, and strategic clarity, they not only fulfil their legal and professional responsibilities but also catalyse a culture rooted in trust and continuous learning. This culture, where openness is not feared but embraced, fosters environments where patient safety thrives, reputations are resilient, and healthcare delivery evolves with integrity. For clinicians and managers alike, mastering these communication strategies is a profound investment in professional confidence and, most importantly, in the well-being of the patients they serve.

Learning from Harm: Investigations and Improvement

Conducting Effective Investigations

When an unexpected adverse event unfolds within a healthcare setting, the instinctive response often carries emotional weight, confusion, urgency and sometimes even fear. Yet beneath these immediate reactions lies the imperative to conduct an investigation that is fair, methodical, and geared toward genuine learning rather than casting blame. Effectively investigating incidents is central to fulfilling the Duty of Candour, as it not only honours the truth of what happened but also paves the way for safer healthcare delivery in the future. Rooted in principles of transparency, respect, and systemic inquiry, the investigative process demands a careful balance: it must be thorough enough to reveal underlying causes without alienating or intimidating those involved. This delicate interplay of fairness and rigor creates a foundation on which healthcare organisations can build resilience and improved safety cultures.

A fundamental principle guiding effective investigations is the clear understanding that errors rarely arise from a single individual's failure; rather, they are often the culminating result of complex interactions within systems, processes, and human factors. This systemic perspective shifts focus away from redundancy and punitive mindsets, redirecting energy towards unearthing vulnerabilities embedded within processes and environments that allowed harm to occur. By adopting this approach, investigations become powerful tools for change, unearthing root causes that might otherwise remain hidden and vulnerable to repetition if left unaddressed. It is imperative, therefore, to foster a mindset that views investigations as learning opportunities rather than fault-finding missions, encouraging open participation from all stakeholders without fear of retribution.

The first step in conducting a meaningful investigation is assembling a balanced, competent team that can approach the incident from multiple perspectives. Including clinicians who were directly involved, alongside impartial professionals such as quality and safety experts, managers, and, when appropriate, patient representatives, enriches the investigation with diverse viewpoints. This collaborative approach promotes comprehensiveness by allowing cross-disciplinary insights into the sequence of events and contributing factors. Importantly, team members should be trained in investigative techniques and understand the goals of the inquiry, safeguarding consistent methodologies and minimising biases that might skew findings. Involving those who are familiar with the operational realities ensures a nuanced understanding, while fresh eyes help identify assumptions that insiders might overlook.

Taking a systematic and structured approach to data collection is vital. This process begins with gathering all relevant information related to the event, including clinical records, communication logs, equipment maintenance reports, and timelines. Conducting interviews is often pivotal in this phase. These should be carried out in an environment that is non-threatening and emphasises psychological safety to encourage candidness. Skilled interviewers employ open-ended questions that allow individuals to narrate their experience freely, rather than constraining them with narrowly focused queries. This technique often reveals critical nuances, such as the subtle decisions, environmental distractions, or resource limitations that standard documentation may omit. It's important to recognise that people's recollections may differ, and discrepancies must be viewed not as contradictions but as complementary pieces that, when combined thoughtfully, provide a fuller picture.

Once sufficient data is collected, the subsequent step involves methodical analysis aimed at identifying root causes and contributory factors. Several techniques are valuable in this endeavour, such as root cause analysis (RCA), failure mode and effects analysis (FMEA), and the five whys method. RCA is particularly prominent in healthcare investigations as it guides inquiry beyond proximate, superficial errors to explore underlying latent conditions that shape behaviour and decision-making. For example, an apparent medication error might trace back to ambiguous labelling practices, understaffing, or failures in the electronic prescribing system. The analytical process involves dissecting the timeline of the incident, reconstructing workflows, and mapping interactions between human and technological elements. Importantly, identifying root causes is not a purely technical exercise; it requires reflective judgement informed by clinical expertise, organisational knowledge, and awareness of human factors.

Throughout the analysis, it is crucial to maintain a transparent narrative that connects factual findings with context, avoiding oversimplification or assigning blame to individuals. Root cause identification should be communicated in a way that fosters shared understanding among all stakeholders, including patients and families affected by the incident. This candid approach respects their right to know and actively involves them in the journey toward learning and improvement. Transparency here does not equate to divulging all raw data indiscriminately but rather to presenting clear, truthful explanations that acknowledge harm while emphasising corrective actions underway.

A cornerstone of translating investigative findings into meaningful change lies in the development and implementation of targeted recommendations. These should be specific, actionable, and measurable, leaving no ambiguity about what needs to be done, who is responsible, and within what timeframe. Moreover, recommendations ought to be prioritised based on potential impact and feasibility, recognising organisational capacities and resource constraints. For instance, a recommendation to enhance electronic health record interfaces might require phased investments, staff training, and iterative feedback loops to be effective. Equally important is the inclusion of strategies that address both technical fixes, such as updating protocols or equipment and cultural improvements like boosting communication or teamwork. By addressing the technical and human dimensions simultaneously, organisations strengthen their resilience against future errors.

Monitoring and follow-up are often overlooked but vital components of the investigative continuum. Simply making recommendations is insufficient; consistent review of progress ensures changes are embedded and produce the intended effect. Establishing clear metrics and regular reporting timelines helps keep improvement efforts on track and accountable. Leaders should foster an environment that values continuous monitoring, encouraging staff to remain vigilant for any signs that risks persist or new challenges have emerged. This commitment to sustained oversight reinforces the learning cycle, signalling that investigations are not isolated responses but ongoing investments in patient safety.

Investigative work must also acknowledge the emotional and psychological impacts on healthcare staff involved in adverse events. Investigations can evoke feelings of guilt, anxiety, and isolation, which, if unaddressed, may inhibit openness and learning. Cultivating a just culture, where staff are supported rather than punished except in cases of recklessness or intent, enables more truthful self-reporting and frank discussions. Providing access to counselling or peer support resources during and after investigations is essential to maintain workforce wellbeing. When clinicians feel valued and protected, their engagement enhances the depth and quality of investigations, benefitting the entire safety ecosystem.

Technology increasingly plays a supportive role in investigations by enabling the collection and analysis of vast amounts of data quickly and accurately. Incident reporting systems, electronic health records, and data analytics tools can uncover patterns or clusters of harm that might be invisible in isolated cases. However, reliance on technology alone is insufficient. The interpretation of data remains a nuanced task requiring human judgement to integrate contextual factors and ethical considerations. Investigators must remain vigilant to the potential pitfalls of overdependence on automated findings, ensuring that technology augments rather than replaces thoughtful inquiry.

To ensure investigations truly advance the Duty of Candour, communication with patients and families must be woven into every stage of the process. Early engagement, when appropriate, helps establish trust and demonstrates organisational commitment to openness. Keeping affected individuals informed of investigation progress, findings, and remedial actions respects their dignity and agency. It also provides opportunities for patients and families to contribute their insights, which may reveal overlooked elements and enrich the investigation. This partnership approach transforms adverse events from solely tragic occurrences into collaborative learning moments, strengthening the patient-clinician relationship despite difficult circumstances.

Finally, a reflective stance is indispensable to every effective investigation. Rather than viewing incidents as isolated misfortunes, healthcare professionals and organisations must embrace the inherent complexity of care delivery. This involves continuously questioning assumptions, recognising the limitations of prior knowledge, and adapting to evolving contexts. Every investigation is an invitation to deepen understanding of the systems and cultures we operate within, and to innovate ways of delivering safer, more compassionate care. Embedding this ethos into routine practice ensures that the Duty of Candour transcends regulatory compliance, emerging as a lived value across all levels of healthcare.

In conclusion, conducting effective investigations after adverse events demands an integrated, compassionate, and methodical approach. By assembling multidisciplinary teams, gathering comprehensive data sensitively, applying rigorous root cause analyses, developing actionable improvements, and maintaining ongoing monitoring, healthcare organisations can transform adversity into opportunity. Supporting the emotional well-being of staff and engaging patients throughout the process further strengthens trust and learning. Leveraging technology thoughtfully and upholding a culture of reflection completes the picture, fostering environments where candour is not feared but embraced. Through such dedicated effort, investigations shine as vital mechanisms not merely for unravelling what went wrong but for illuminating pathways to safer, more transparent healthcare futures.

Identifying Systemic Issues

In the complex web of healthcare delivery, when an adverse event occurs, it is all too tempting to focus on individual errors, the missteps, oversights, or lapses in judgment that often appear as the immediate causes of harm. Yet, transformed by decades of patient safety scholarship and practical experience, contemporary understanding urges us to look far beyond the surface level of frontline errors and to uncover the deeper, often hidden, systemic factors that shape the conditions in which care is provided. Identifying these systemic issues is not merely an academic exercise but a vital step toward instigating meaningful, sustainable change that can prevent recurrence of similar events. It is an act of humility, recognising that even the most diligent and skilled healthcare professional operates within an environment shaped by tools, policies, workflows, leadership decisions, culture, and resource constraints. This systemic lens fosters investigations that are balanced, fair, and ultimately constructive, diffusing the blame culture that can cripple openness and learning.

At the heart of identifying systemic issues lies an understanding that errors rarely occur in isolation. Individual mistakes are often the tip of a much larger iceberg composed of latent conditions within the healthcare system. These latent conditions, embedded in organisational design, procedures, technology interfaces, and cultural norms, lie dormant and unrecognised until they interact with triggering events under particular circumstances. To pursue root causes that permit systemic learning requires a shift from a punitive mindset to a questioning, analytical approach that rigorously interrogates how the design and functioning of the entire system contributed to the outcome. For example, rather than concluding that a nurse's failure to double-check a medication dose was simply carelessness, a systemic inquiry might explore whether overloaded staffing, rushed workflows, unclear labelling, or poorly designed electronic medication administration records created an environment where errors could more readily occur. Each of these systemic factors can either pave the way for error or serve as a barrier that prevents it from reaching the patient. Untangling these interwoven elements demands a commitment to holistic investigation that goes beyond assigning individual fault.

One of the most valuable methodologies to uncover these systemic factors is the root cause analysis (RCA). Unlike traditional investigations that might stop at the 'who' and 'what' of an incident, RCA delves into the 'why' and 'how.' It systematically probes the contributing elements at multiple layers within the system. This process often begins by mapping the sequence of events leading up to the adverse outcome, guided by those directly involved, to ensure an accurate and detailed narrative. By gently interviewing front-line staff, managers, and even patients or families where appropriate, investigators collect diverse perspectives that shed light on weaknesses and tensions in the care delivery process. The RCA further explores human factors, environmental conditions, communication breakdowns, training deficits, equipment usability, and organisational policies that influenced behaviours and decision-making. Through iterative questioning, such as "why did this happen?" repeated multiple times, root causes unfold like the rings of a tree, revealing fundamental flaws in the system rather than proximal errors alone.

It is essential to recognise that organisations are complicated adaptive systems where many interdependent components interplay in dynamic and sometimes unpredictable ways. Therefore, the pursuit of identifying systemic issues must maintain an openness to complexity rather than seeking simplistic linear chains of causation. Often, multiple contributing factors combine synergistically to trigger adverse events, including technology design that interferes with workflows, hierarchical communication barriers that obstruct concerns from being voiced, inadequate supervision, or competing priorities imposed by demanding performance targets. Investigations must uncover these entanglements, understanding that no single element is solely to blame but rather that the confluence of several insufficiencies forms a perfect storm. When this perspective is embedded in the investigation culture, it encourages a learning orientation that accepts complexity and nuance instead of reductionist blame-seeking.

A powerful tool in this endeavour is the systems thinking approach, which encourages investigators and healthcare leaders to view care processes as interconnected wholes rather than isolated tasks. Systems thinking goes beyond root cause analysis by integrating feedback loops and recognising the dynamic interactions within and between teams, departments, and organisational layers. For example, a medication error that occurred at bedside might reflect upstream issues such as formulary restrictions imposed by pharmacy, delayed transmission of laboratory results, or software interface confusion across digital platforms. Systems thinking facilitates a broader mapping of these connections and reveals where systemic bottlenecks or incompatible designs are undermining patient safety. This approach equips organisations to transition from reactive incident management toward proactive system redesign, emphasising resilience and adaptability. Embracing this perspective means that rather than seeking scapegoats, attention is devoted to building system defences, redundancies, and buffers that protect patients despite inevitable human fallibility.

However, identifying systemic problems is not just about technical analysis; it also demands cultural introspection. The environment in which healthcare professionals work profoundly influences whether systemic issues can be identified and acknowledged openly. In settings where blame is swiftly assigned, and professionals fear repercussions, silence and concealment often protect flawed system designs from scrutiny. To break this cycle, organisations must foster psychological safety and an atmosphere where all members feel empowered and supported to voice concerns, report errors, and participate in investigations without fear of stigma or punishment. Encouraging open dialogue about systemic vulnerabilities requires leaders who exemplify humility and curiosity rather than defensiveness. Frontline staff who bear the brunt of system failures must be treated as partners in safety improvement, their insights valued as crucial data points rather than grounds for reprimand. When psychological safety is in place, the identification of systemic weaknesses becomes a shared mission, enriched by collective wisdom rather than stifled by hierarchy and blame.

Once systemic issues have been identified, the challenge shifts toward translating these insights into effective organisational changes that reduce risk and enhance care quality. This requires a disciplined and iterative approach where recommendations are carefully designed to address root system flaws, not just symptoms. Interventions could range from revising protocols and workflows, upgrading or replacing equipment, enhancing training programs, adjusting staffing models, improving communication channels, or redesigning physical spaces. Importantly, change initiatives must be monitored and evaluated continuously to verify that they achieve intended outcomes and do not introduce new risks. This commitment to monitoring creates a learning loop that strengthens organisational resilience. Establishing multidisciplinary safety committees that include clinicians, managers, risk experts, and patient representatives can facilitate this oversight, ensuring that changes are responsive, well-coordinated, and grounded in front-line reality.

Equally vital is the role of data in identifying systemic issues and informing improvements. Trends in incident reports, near misses, complaints, and safety audits provide a rich reservoir of information that can highlight patterns pointing to systemic weaknesses. For instance, repeated delays in discharge processing or medication administration errors may indicate systemic flaws in communication tools or workload distribution. However, data collection alone is insufficient if it is not analysed with a systems lens and integrated into decision-making frameworks that prioritise safety culture. Healthcare organisations that succeed in this endeavour develop transparent reporting mechanisms and feedback loops that make safety data understandable and actionable for all staff levels. Moreover, involving patients and families in reporting and investigation processes can reveal systemic gaps that may be invisible to professionals, such as cultural insensitivity, fragmented care coordination, or information barriers. Their lived experience adds an irreplaceable dimension to system analysis.

In practical terms, conducting investigations focused on systemic learning rather than blame demands skilled facilitation and clear processes. Teams charged with incident review must be trained not only in technical investigation methods but also in human factors and communication skills that elicit honest input from participants. Investigators should guard against cognitive biases that can cloud judgment, such as confirmation bias, only seeing factors that support preconceived notions or outcome bias, judging decisions solely by their result rather than the conditions under which they were made. Maintaining neutrality and curiosity in the investigative process encourages richer data collection and a more nuanced understanding of systemic vulnerabilities. Transparency about investigation goals to learn and improve rather than to penalise must be communicated clearly to all involved, fostering trust and cooperation.

It is also crucial to appreciate that system improvement is not a one-off event but a continuous journey. Healthcare systems evolve constantly, with new technologies, policies, and workforce changes altering risk profiles daily. Therefore, the identification of systemic issues and subsequent remedial actions requires ongoing vigilance and agility. Cultivating a culture of continuous improvement involves regular reassessment of system performance, openness to innovation, and candid reflection on failures and successes alike. Successful organisations embed these principles into their governance structures, making safety and quality integral to strategic planning. Leadership commitment at all levels reinforces this ethos and ensures the allocation of resources necessary for meaningful system reforms.

In sum, looking beyond individual errors to identify systemic issues transforms incident response from a culture of fear to a culture of learning and safety enhancement. It respects the complexity of healthcare delivery and acknowledges that improving patient safety is a collective responsibility requiring systemic insight, meaningful engagement, and sustained action. By embracing rigorous investigation methodologies, fostering psychological safety, leveraging data thoughtfully, and committing to continuous improvement, healthcare organisations can convert adverse events into powerful catalysts for positive change. Such a systems-oriented approach ultimately protects not only individual patients but also the integrity and resilience of the entire healthcare enterprise, making openness and accountability foundational rather than adversarial. This shift from blame to learning epitomises the true spirit of practising the duty of candour with confidence.

Implementing and Sustaining Improvements

The task of implementing and sustaining improvements following an adverse event or critical incident within healthcare settings necessitates an intricate balance of rigor, nuance, and sensitivity. At its core, this process is about translating the insights gained from thorough investigations into meaningful, lasting change, a task that demands not only clinical acumen but also sophisticated change management strategies infused with empathy and organisational savvy. The endeavour begins with the recognition that the primary goal of any post-incident investigation is to foster a culture of learning and safety rather than blame or punishment. This foundational mindset is critical, as it shapes the receptivity of all stakeholders to forthcoming changes and their commitment to embedding these reforms into the everyday fabric of care delivery.

Effective change management within this context requires that leaders and clinical teams alike approach improvements with a strategic lens that appreciates both the human and systemic dimensions of healthcare. Change rarely occurs in isolation; it ripples through complex networks of relationships, routines, professional identities, and institutional norms. Therefore, to implement improvements successfully, leaders must engage in stakeholder analysis, pinpointing who will be most affected by changes, who must support them for success, and who might resist. Often, resistance stems from understandable apprehensions about increased workload, loss of autonomy, or fear of scrutiny. Addressing these concerns transparently, listening actively to feedback, and co-creating solutions with frontline staff fosters a sense of ownership and shared responsibility, thereby breaking down barriers that commonly derail change efforts.

A vital component of this journey lies in articulating a clear and compelling rationale for change. When healthcare professionals, managers, and support staff understand the 'why' behind new procedures rooted firmly in both patient safety imperatives and ethical obligations, they are far more likely to commit emotionally and intellectually. Storytelling is a potent tool in this regard; weaving narratives around real incidents, their impact on patients and families, and the lessons drawn can help transform abstract policies into tangible human commitments. Equally important is framing improvements as opportunities for professional growth and enhanced patient-centred care, appealing to deeply held values that motivate healthcare workers daily.

Once consensus and commitment begin to coalesce, the execution phase demands careful planning and resource allocation. Change initiatives must be broken down into achievable, sequenced steps, each with clearly defined objectives, roles, and timelines. This prevents staff overwhelm and ensures that momentum is maintained. Integration of new practices into existing workflows is crucial; sudden, dramatic shifts can disrupt care continuity and provoke anxiety. Therefore, iterative pilot testing within smaller units or teams allows for fine-tuning adaptations, gathering real-world feedback, and mitigating unforeseen consequences. These pilots also serve as proof of concept, showcasing early successes that reinforce confidence and sustain enthusiasm.

Robust training and education efforts are indispensable in equipping all involved personnel with the knowledge, skills, and attitudes needed to enact improvements confidently. This includes not only formal sessions but also a culture of ongoing learning, where questions, concerns, and suggestions are welcomed continuously. Multimodal educational approaches combining didactic teaching, simulation exercises, reflective practice, and peer mentoring help accommodate diverse learning styles and embed new competencies more deeply. Leaders who model vulnerability and openness during this phase, openly sharing their own reflections on the learning process, foster psychological safety that encourages widespread engagement.

Sustaining improvements over time is arguably the greatest challenge, as initial enthusiasm often wanes when faced with the daily pressures and competing priorities typical of healthcare environments. To counteract this, embedding monitoring and feedback mechanisms is a critical strategy. Clear metrics aligned to the desired outcomes should be established early and tracked systematically, providing objective data on whether changes are being implemented as planned and if they are achieving intended safety gains. Regular feedback loops where data is shared transparently with staff not only maintain awareness but also enable rapid identification of areas needing reinforcement or adjustment. When staff see tangible evidence that their efforts are making a difference, motivation and commitment are renewed.

Accountability frameworks must be supportive rather than punitive, focusing on collective responsibility for improvement. This is where leadership plays a pivotal role; leaders must continuously champion the changes, celebrate successes publicly, and act swiftly to address lapses or emerging obstacles. Maintaining open communication channels across hierarchies ensures that frontline insights can inform ongoing refinement, making the improvement process dynamic rather than static. Peer support networks and communities of practice provide additional scaffolding, enabling healthcare professionals to share experiences, troubleshoot challenges, and propagate best practices collaboratively.

The organisational culture profoundly influences both the implementation and sustenance of improvements. Cultivating a culture that normalises reflection, inquiry, and candour hinges on trust that raising concerns will lead to constructive action, not retribution; trust that leadership values transparency; trust that patients' voices are honoured. Leaders committed to nurturing such a culture invest time and attention in building relationships, demonstrating empathy, and consistently modelling the behaviours they expect. Recognition and reward systems attuned to supporting openness and learning fortify these cultural shifts, signalling organisational priorities unequivocally.

Moreover, the nuances of healthcare settings varying by size, specialty, resources, and local context require that change strategies be adaptable and sensitive to unique circumstances. For instance, rural or resource-limited environments may necessitate creative solutions that leverage existing strengths and networks, while large academic centres might focus on integrating technological tools for data capture and communication. Embracing diversity in solutions and encouraging innovation prevents a one-size-fits-all approach that risks alienating teams or failing to capture the complexity of clinical realities.

Equally integral to sustaining improvements is the alignment of external regulatory expectations with internal organisational goals. Healthcare organisations must remain vigilant about emerging regulatory standards related to the duty of candour and safety reporting. Proactively engaging with regulators as partners, rather than adversaries, can provide additional impetus and resources for continuous improvement. This symbiotic relationship also aids in harmonising policies, ensuring compliance, and fostering credibility with patients and the broader public.

One cannot underestimate the emotional labour that accompanies implementing changes after adverse incidents. Healthcare professionals often experience moral distress, guilt, and anxiety that can impair their ability to engage fully with improvement efforts. Addressing these emotional dimensions through structured support such as debriefings, counselling services, and peer support is essential. When staff feel cared for and psychologically safe, they are better equipped to participate constructively and sustain behavioural changes over time.

Technology also presents both challenges and opportunities for change management. Electronic health records, incident reporting systems, and communication platforms can streamline information flow and increase transparency. However, the introduction of technological solutions must be carefully managed to avoid unintended consequences such as information overload, workflow disruption, or depersonalisation of communication. Inclusive user involvement in the design and rollout of these tools is paramount to align functionality with real-world needs and enhance acceptance.

In reflecting upon the multifaceted challenge of implementing and sustaining improvements, it becomes clear that success is not merely a product of good intentions or isolated interventions. Instead, it emerges from a coherent, intentional orchestration of leadership vision, strategic planning, inclusive engagement, ongoing education, data-informed feedback, emotional support, and an unwavering commitment to patient-centred values. When these elements converge, healthcare organisations can transform the aftermath of harm into fertile ground for resilience, learning, and enhanced care quality.

Ultimately, the narrative of change management in this context is a story about human connection and systemic evolution intertwined. It recognises that healthcare professionals, managers, patients, and families are co-authors of safer, more transparent care, bound by the shared responsibility to learn from mistakes and strive ceaselessly for improvement. By approaching implementation with humility, patience, and persistence, organisations not only fulfil their duty of candour but elevate the very essence of compassionate healthcare delivery, crafting environments where honesty, trust, and progress are not exceptions but the celebrated norm.

Building a Culture of Openness: Leadership and Teamwork

Leadership Commitment to Candour

Leadership commitment to candour is the cornerstone upon which an entire culture of transparency and trust is built within healthcare organisations. It is not merely a matter of issuing statements or policies mandating honesty when things go wrong; rather, it hinges on leaders embodying the principles of candour in their daily actions, decisions, and communication. When those at the helm of healthcare institutions openly embrace candour, they set an unequivocal tone that resonates throughout every level of the organisation, sending a powerful message that honesty is not only expected but respected and rewarded. This tone from the top is integral for cultivating an environment where psychological safety flourishes, where clinicians, managers, and staff feel confident to speak up, disclose errors, and engage in candid conversations without fear of blame or retribution. In this way, the commitment displayed by leaders becomes the blueprint for how candour permeates clinical practice, governance, and patient interactions.

To genuinely model candour, leaders must adopt a stance of vulnerability and accountability themselves. It is not enough to profess the virtues of openness; they must demonstrate it in moments of challenge and uncertainty. This involves acknowledging when mistakes are made in leadership or when policies fail to protect patients adequately. The courage displayed in admitting one's own fallibility serves as a powerful catalyst, inviting others to follow suit. Leadership's willingness to discuss shortcomings transparently amidst pressures of institutional reputation and public scrutiny signals that candour is a shared responsibility, irrespective of hierarchy or role. This modelling sustains authenticity, dispels the toxic myths about the inevitability of punitive consequences, and nurtures trust, which is the lifeblood of effective communication and patient safety.

A pivotal element in embedding candour within organisational culture lies in the conscious and consistent promotion of psychological safety. Leaders play an indispensable role in creating and maintaining environments where staff feel safe to voice concerns, report incidents, and admit errors without fear of humiliation or job loss. This is a profound shift from traditional approaches that prioritise blame and discipline, which often stifle openness and risk concealment of harm. Achieving psychological safety demands deliberate actions: leaders must foster respectful dialogue even in stressful situations, normalise learning from mistakes, and highlight the shared goal of patient well-being over individual fault. Leaders who actively listen, respond constructively to difficult disclosures, and reinforce confidentiality where appropriate, cultivate confidence among colleagues that raising issues will lead to improvements and support, not punishment. Psychological safety thus becomes the fertile soil in which the seeds of candour grow robustly.

Embedding candour into an organisation's DNA also requires leaders to champion educational and training initiatives that hone the skills necessary for candid and compassionate communication.

The art of disclosure, particularly after adverse events, is nuanced and challenging, demanding not only knowledge of legal and ethical obligations but also empathy, emotional intelligence, and cultural sensitivity. Leadership commitment is evidenced by allocating sufficient resources to equip all staff, from frontline clinicians to senior managers, with tailored training that builds competence and confidence in difficult conversations. These trainings should be iterative and dynamic, incorporating real-world scenarios, role-playing, and feedback mechanisms to mirror the complexities encountered in practice. Moreover, leadership involvement in such programs, whether through participation, advocacy, or evaluation, signals prioritisation of candour as a non-negotiable aspect of professional development. The resulting proficiency among staff exponentially enhances the likelihood of timely, truthful, and sensitive disclosures to patients and families, thereby fulfilling the duty of candour with integrity.

Beyond training, leaders must ensure that policies and procedures within the organisation explicitly reflect and support the principles of candour. These frameworks should articulate clear expectations for disclosure, outline processes for managing adverse events transparently, and delineate responsibilities at every level. However, these documents in isolation are insufficient unless leadership actively fosters an environment in which policies are interpreted with a spirit of openness rather than strict compliance or risk avoidance. Leaders should champion ongoing policy review and refinement, incorporating feedback from frontline teams, patients, and external expert bodies. By positioning these policies as living instruments designed to empower transparent communication and learning, leaders demonstrate their commitment to continuous quality improvement. They must also ensure that policies align with broader legal and regulatory frameworks, while being adaptable to the unique cultural context of their organisation, thereby reinforcing candour not as a bureaucratic mandate but as a shared ethical imperative.

Effective communication practices modelled and reinforced by leadership are another key mechanism for embedding candour deeply within healthcare institutions. The language leaders use in meetings, public statements, and informal interactions matters profoundly as it shapes collective attitudes and expectations. Leaders who consistently speak candidly about challenges, openly share lessons learned from errors, and emphasise the human side of care create an organisational narrative anchored in transparency. This does not mean broadcasting every setback indiscriminately but rather framing disclosure as a constructive, compassionate process cantered on restoration and improvement. Crucially, leaders must balance honesty with respect for patient privacy and sensitivity to emotional distress, modelling the fine judgment required to navigate these conversations thoughtfully. Leadership communication also involves recognising and celebrating instances where candour led to meaningful change or strengthened patient relationships. Such positive reinforcement integrates openness into the organisation's identity and motivates ongoing commitment from all team members.

The role of leadership in supporting teams through the emotional and practical challenges of candour cannot be overstated. Adverse events and their disclosure often provoke intense feelings of guilt, fear, grief, or isolation among healthcare professionals. Leaders who anticipate and address these emotional dimensions actively contribute to the resilience and sustainability of candour practices. This support may involve ensuring access to counselling services, peer support programs, and debriefing sessions that create safe spaces for staff to process their experiences. Leaders must be skilled at recognising signs of distress and intervening sensitively to prevent burnout or withdrawal. In addition to emotional support, practical assistance in navigating complex disclosure processes, managing legal implications, and coordinating with multidisciplinary teams is essential. By providing clear guidance, resources, and a nonjudgmental presence, leaders equip their teams to uphold candour without feeling overwhelmed or exposed, reinforcing a cohesive and courageous workforce.

Leadership commitment to candour also requires an outward focus, engaging with patients, families, and external stakeholders transparently and empathetically. When healthcare leaders openly acknowledge incidents, participate in dialogue with affected individuals, and demonstrate genuine accountability on behalf of their organisations, they foster trust that extends beyond institutional walls. This external candour helps rebuild fractured relationships, mitigates reputational damage, and aligns organisational values with societal expectations. Leaders must balance transparency with prudence, ensuring that communication is timely, accurate, and framed within a context of meaningful remedial action and continued learning. Engaging patient and family representatives in policy development and quality improvement initiatives further embeds candour as a collective, inclusive endeavour. This collaborative leadership style transforms the duty of candour from a regulatory obligation into a platform for healing, partnership, and shared responsibility.

Sustaining leadership commitment to candour over time demands ongoing reflection, accountability, and adaptability. Leaders should regularly evaluate the organisational climate regarding transparency, using qualitative and quantitative methods such as staff surveys, incident analysis, and patient feedback. These data illuminate strengths and areas requiring intensified focus, enabling targeted interventions. Importantly, leaders should be prepared to confront uncomfortable truths revealed through such reflections, demonstrating humility and openness to change. Governance mechanisms must include candour as a key performance indicator, embedding transparency within strategic priorities and resource allocation. Continuity of leadership vision is crucial; transitions in leadership roles should preserve and build upon established commitments rather than erode them. Cultivating a pipeline of future leaders who embrace candour principles ensures that the cultural transformation is not ephemeral but enduring. This long-term stewardship is essential to realise the profound patient and organisational benefits that candour promises.

In sum, leadership commitment to candour is not an abstract ideal but a tangible, dynamic process enacted daily through words, actions, policies, and emotional intelligence. Leaders set the cultural tone, create the psychological safety necessary for openness, provide essential training, embed robust policies, model transparent communication, and support their teams emotionally and operationally. They extend candour beyond their institutions by engaging patients and the wider community authentically. Their steadfast stewardship ensures that candour evolves from a regulatory box-ticking exercise into a living, breathing ethos that enhances patient safety, nurtures trust, and drives continuous improvement. In these ways, leaders wield profound influence in transforming the duty of candour from obligation into opportunity, illuminating a path toward a more humane, just, and transparent healthcare system.

Training and Supporting Teams

Building skills and resilience within healthcare teams is an essential cornerstone in nurturing a culture rooted in the Duty of Candour. When leaders commit to supporting their teams rigorously through education, training, and emotional reinforcement, they do more than just comply with policy; they transform the very atmosphere of care, busy hospital wards, community clinics, and specialised units into places where transparency, trust, and compassion become default modes of interaction. Fostering this transformation requires a nuanced understanding that the Duty of Candour is not simply about procedural adherence, but rather about cultivating human connection and moral courage amidst often distressing and complex situations. Teams operating in healthcare are regularly confronting high-stakes environments where mistakes or unexpected outcomes disrupt lives profoundly. Therefore, empowering healthcare professionals to face these challenges with honesty and openness necessitates more than theoretical knowledge; it demands robust, sustained skill-building, bolstered by an environment that prioritises psychological safety and resilience.

Effective training programs for teams practicing candour must reach beyond simple awareness campaigns or checklists. They should immerse clinicians and healthcare workers in scenarios that simulate real-life adverse events, encouraging reflective learning and empathy. Role-play exercises, carefully constructed to mirror sensitive conversations with patients and families, allow participants to practice the delicate art of truth-telling infused with compassion. Within these simulated dialogues, healthcare providers can safely engage with difficult emotions, fear, guilt, grief and experience firsthand the profound impact of words chosen and withheld. Such experiential learning not only enhances communication skills but also deepens emotional intelligence, enabling professionals to respond to patients' distress with authenticity and grace. Leaders who design and champion these training initiatives recognise that candour is as much an emotional journey as it is a procedural one and that preparing teams means to prepare hearts as well as minds.

Psychological safety, a vital underpinning for open communication, must be woven into every thread of the healthcare culture. When team members trust that they can speak up about errors or near misses without retribution or humiliation, the organisation unlocks a wealth of knowledge critical to patient safety. Leaders play a pivotal role here: they must consistently demonstrate vulnerability by acknowledging their own mistakes and uncertainties, thus modelling that error is a human experience and an opportunity for growth rather than a cause for shame. This leadership behaviour cascades through hierarchical layers, gradually dismantling barriers that inhibit honest discussion and creating an environment where every voice, from junior nurses to senior consultants, feels valued and protected. Consequently, staff are more likely to report incidents promptly, engage in meaningful dialogue about improvement measures, and internalise the principles of the Duty of Candour as integral to their professional identity rather than as an external imposition.

Beyond formal training, ongoing support structures are crucial to sustain resilience among healthcare teams practicing candour. Harmful incidents, by their nature, inflict emotional trauma not only on patients and families but also on the clinicians involved, often referred to as the "second victims." Leaders must ensure that mechanisms such as peer support programs, confidential counselling services, and debriefing sessions are readily accessible and actively promoted. These resources help mitigate burnout, guilt, and moral distress by providing safe spaces for reflection and emotional processing. When individual resilience is nurtured at the organisational level, teams collectively strengthen their capacity to handle adversity with composure and ethical integrity. This resilience undergirds a culture where openness about mistakes is not perceived as personal failure but rather as responsible professionalism dedicated to constant learning and patient welfare.

Communication practices promulgated through training must explicitly include how to navigate the complex dynamics of disclosing incidents truthfully while preserving respect and dignity for all parties involved. Skills such as active listening, non-verbal cue recognition, and empathetic phrasing are essential tools that require deliberate cultivation. Leaders must encourage feedback loops where team members observe and critique communication styles constructively, fostering continuous improvement. Additionally, training should address common fears that inhibit candour, fear of blame, litigation, or damage to reputation by clarifying legal protections and organisational policies that support disclosure. Understanding that apologising and admitting error do not automatically invite punitive consequences reassures clinicians and emboldens them to engage openly. When healthcare professionals internalise this knowledge, they move from defensive silence to courageous transparency, shifting the organisation's narrative around harm.

Embedding candour into policies and procedures is another aspect of fostering skills and resilience, acting as a compass to guide behaviours consistently across varied clinical settings. Policies outlining exact steps for disclosure, timelines, and documentation create clarity and reduce ambiguity in stressful moments. Training must include thorough familiarisation with these policies to ensure that teams not only understand expectations but also feel competent in applying them practically. When policies are integrated seamlessly into everyday workflows and supported by technological tools like electronic incident reporting systems, the act of candour becomes less daunting and more routine. Leaders have a responsibility to review and revise policies regularly, incorporating frontline feedback and emerging best practices, thus demonstrating that the duty of candour is a living, evolving standard rather than a static, bureaucratic checklist.

Moreover, leadership commitment to visible and sustained reinforcement of candour practices has a profound influence on team morale and engagement. Regular meetings, newsletters, and informal conversations that highlight candour success stories, acknowledge the courage of staff who disclose incidents, and share lessons learned, reinforce positive behaviours. Celebrating transparency publicly signals organisational values and encourages others to emulate these practices, creating a virtuous cycle of openness and improvement. Leaders who foster such narratives help dismantle the stigma surrounding errors and urge teams to view these moments as pivotal turning points for systemic change rather than occasions for punishment.

In addition, training initiatives should be tailored to the diverse roles, experiences, and cultural backgrounds of healthcare team members. Recognising that the needs and challenges facing a junior nurse in an emergency department differ markedly from those of a senior surgeon or allied health professional working in a rehabilitation setting is essential for crafting relevant, engaging education. Training delivered in a culturally competent manner respects linguistic nuances, communication preferences, and varying perceptions of authority and harm. Inclusive approaches encourage all team members to participate fully and contribute their unique perspectives to building a comprehensive understanding and practice of candour. When teams feel seen and respected in their diversity, their commitment to transparency deepens, and organisational resilience to incidents strengthens.

The integration of technology and digital platforms also represents a valuable frontier in training and supporting healthcare teams. Simulation software, virtual reality, and e-learning modules facilitate flexible and immersive learning experiences that accommodate the often-unpredictable schedules of clinical staff. These tools can replicate the emotional intensity of disclosure conversations and allow repeated practice without risk, fostering confidence and competence. Digital platforms also offer opportunities for peer-to-peer learning and sharing of best practices across departments and institutions, spreading the culture of candour beyond local silos. Leaders who invest in these innovations demonstrate adaptive and forward-thinking stewardship of their teams' development, signalling that commitment to candour evolves alongside advances in education technology.

Finally, the ongoing evaluation of training effectiveness and team support mechanisms is indispensable to ensure that capacity-building efforts translate into meaningful changes in practice. Measures might include surveys assessing staff comfort with disclosure, audits of incident reporting compliance, and qualitative feedback from patients and families regarding their experiences of candour. Leaders must establish systems to gather and analyse these data regularly, using findings to refine training programs and support offerings dynamically. This reflective process maintains momentum and accountability, ensuring that skills and resilience do not erode over time. The ultimate goal is that every team member feels equipped and empowered to uphold the Duty of Candour steadfastly, not merely in theory, but through consistent, confident action that honours the dignity and safety of those entrusted to their care.

In summary, building skills and resilience in healthcare teams for practising the Duty of Candour demands a multi-faceted and deeply human approach. It requires immersive, empathetic training that goes beyond policy recitation to develop communication prowess and emotional intelligence. It calls for leadership that models vulnerability and fosters psychological safety, nurturing environments where openness can flourish unencumbered by fear. Continuous support through peer networks and mental health resources fortifies professionals against the strains of disclosure, while clear, accessible policies provide the structural framework for consistent practice. Tailored, culturally sensitive education, amplified through digital innovations, ensures inclusivity and flexibility, appealing to the rich diversity within healthcare teams. Rigorous evaluation and feedback loops maintain integrity and growth in these efforts over time. Through these integrated strategies, healthcare organisations can embed candour not just as an obligation to fulfil but as a shared, resilient strength that enhances trust, learning, and compassionate care for all.

Policy Development and Communication

In the intricate tapestry of healthcare organisations, policy development and communication form the warp and weft that hold the fabric of openness and candour together. Embedding a culture of transparency requires more than well-intentioned efforts or isolated initiatives; it necessitates the deliberate crafting of robust policies that not only reflect ethical mandates but also resonate meaningfully within the everyday reality of clinical practice. These policies become the scaffolding upon which trust is built, both internally within teams and externally with patients and their families. Yet, the mere existence of a policy document is insufficient. The process through which policies are developed and subsequently communicated determines their efficacy in embedding openness at every level of the organisation.

Leadership must approach policy development as a dynamic and collaborative endeavour rather than a top-down imposition. This means engaging frontline clinicians, managerial staff, patient representatives, and even legal advisors in the initial stages of formulating frameworks governing the duty of candour. When diverse voices contribute to shaping the principles and procedures, the resulting policies are not only more comprehensive but also garner broader ownership and adherence. Collaboration clarifies ambiguities and anticipates practical challenges, allowing policies to be crafted with nuance and relevance, key factors in the translation of abstract ideals into actionable behaviours. This inclusive approach also strengthens psychological safety, as staff realise that the policy is not a punitive script but a supportive guideline created with sensitivity to their realities, fears, and aspirations.

The clarity of language within duty of candour policies is paramount. The temptation to couch policies in dense legal jargon or organisational bureaucracy can alienate those the policy aims to guide. Instead, policies must be written in plain, accessible language that speaks directly to healthcare professionals' values and responsibilities. Articulating the moral imperatives alongside the legal obligations reinforces the understanding that candour is not merely compliance but a commitment to patients and to the integrity of the profession. Moreover, policies should explicitly acknowledge the emotional complexity inherent in admitting mistakes and communicating harm, validating healthcare workers' feelings and promoting self-compassion alongside accountability. This authenticity in wording tends to dismantle defensive postures and encourages a culture where openness is perceived as strength rather than vulnerability.

Equally critical is the framing of duty of candour policies within a larger ecosystem of organisational commitments to quality improvement and patient safety. When candour policies sit in isolation, employees may perceive disclosures as one-off incidents rather than part of a continuous journey toward excellence. Leadership must weave these policies into the broader narrative of safety culture, where learning from harm, no matter how uncomfortable does the organisation treasures an opportunity. This integration helps shift the mindset away from blame and fear toward curiosity and resilience. In doing so, the policy becomes a living document that evolves with each new insight, reflecting the dynamic nature of healthcare delivery and the human experience within it.

Once carefully developed, the communication of these policies is an equally vital endeavour demanding strategic thought and empathetic execution. Deploying a new or revised duty of candour policy should never be relegated to a perfunctory announcement buried in an email or stuck on an intranet page. Instead, leadership must orchestrate a sustained campaign of communication tailored to the multifaceted realities of healthcare teams. This may include interactive workshops, scenario-based learning sessions, and facilitated discussions that encourage dialogue rather than passive reception. Such environments permit questions, address uncertainties, and confront the emotional nuances of disclosure conversations. Embedding storytelling and real-world examples into these communications humanises policy content, making the abstract real and relevant. By sharing narratives of both challenges and successes, organisations signal that they value growth and support, reinforcing psychological safety.

Furthermore, the cadence and channels of policy communication matter profoundly in embedding candour. A single launch event will not suffice; ongoing reinforcement is essential. Integrating reminders about candour policies into regular staff meetings, clinical governance forums, and performance appraisals ensures the ethos remains alive and at the forefront of mind. Visual aids, such as posters and pocket guides, can provide quick references to principles and practical steps. Leadership visibility in these efforts carries symbolic weight; when senior executives and clinical leaders openly champion the principles of candour and visibly engage in communication initiatives, their actions set a potent example that permeates organisational culture. Conversely, policy initiatives risk stagnation without these visible role models to kindle momentum.

In the domain of communication, it is imperative to recognise the diversity within healthcare teams not only in terms of professional roles but also cultural backgrounds, languages, and individual experiences with error and disclosure. Tailoring communication strategies to accommodate this diversity is not merely good practice but foundational to true inclusion and equity. This may include translating policy documents, offer cultural competence training, and adapt communication workshops to reflect different worldviews on error and responsibility. Such sensitivity ensures that all healthcare workers feel seen, heard, and valued in the shared mission of transparency, thereby strengthening adherence and reducing disparities in how candour is practised.

Embedding openness also hinges on supporting healthcare professionals in managing the emotional and practical complexities of candid disclosure. Policies must outline the availability and scope of support mechanisms such as debriefing sessions, counselling services, and peer support networks. Communication about these supports should be proactive and destigmatised, so seeking help after an adverse event becomes normalised rather than taboo. When staff know they are not alone, when leadership openly advocates for their well-being, the psychological safety necessary for authentic candour flourishes. This support infrastructure operates symbiotically with clear policies to create an environment where mistakes are acknowledged openly and addressed constructively rather than concealed through fear.

In addition, to truly embed candour, organisations must consider the myriad interfaces where communication policies intersect. For instance, the relationship with external bodies such as regulators, legal advisers, and patient advocacy groups demands policies that delineate timelines, responsibilities, and modes of disclosure. Staff must understand how their internal disclosure efforts align with these external requirements without fostering defensive or secretive behaviour. Clear internal communication about these intersections demystifies the process and enables healthcare professionals to act consistently and confidently, knowing their disclosures contribute to both organisational accountability and patient trust.

The iterative nature of policy development and communication should be emphasised within organisations. Policies should be living texts that reflect emerging legal frameworks, lessons learned from past incidents, and evolving best practices. Similarly, feedback loops from frontline staff regarding the clarity, relevance, and impact of policies are invaluable. Leadership must establish mechanisms whereby concerns or suggestions about the duty of candour policy can be raised and acted upon transparently. Such responsiveness signals an organisational humility that bolsters faith in institutional commitments to openness. Sharing these developments openly within the organisation further reinforces a culture where learning is prioritised and where policies are not static mandates but evolving partnerships between leadership and the workforce.

Moreover, embedding openness into systems demands alignment between policies and tangible resources. Communication policies must be accompanied by adequate time allowances, staffing provisions, and training investments so that healthcare professionals can practise candour without feeling rushed or unsupported. Without these enablers, even the best-designed policies risk remaining aspirational ideals rather than everyday realities. Leadership plays a crucial role here by advocating for the allocation of resources necessary to sustain candid communication and to embed it meaningfully within clinical workflows. These investments are, ultimately, declarations of value, signalling that transparency and patient-centred care are indeed organisational priorities.

Finally, it is vital to recognise that embedding openness is not merely a procedural exercise but a profound cultural transformation requiring patience, persistence, and passionate leadership. Policies serve as the compass, communication as the beacon, but courage and commitment among healthcare professionals actualise this vision. The journey may encounter resistance rooted in fear, shame, or uncertainty; hence, compassionate leadership that models vulnerability alongside strength becomes a lodestar. Celebrating small victories, instances where candour was practised successfully, lessons were learned, and relationships were strengthened, nurtures hope and momentum. Through thoughtful policy development, empathetic communication, and unwavering leadership support, healthcare organisations can transcend the perception of candour as an imposed obligation and embrace it as an empowering pathway to trust, healing, and enduring patient safety.

Case Studies and Practical Tools

Case Study Analyses

In the intricate world of healthcare, where human lives and unpredictable events entwine, it is often through the lens of real incidents that profound understanding and meaningful learning emerge. The practice of the Duty of Candour, rooted in transparency, empathy, and accountability, finds its fullest expression not in abstract guidelines alone but in the lived experiences of healthcare professionals, patients, and families navigating the turbulent aftermath of unintended harm. It is in these moments, when things go wrong, that the principles underpinning candour are tested, challenged, and ultimately reinforced. This subchapter draws deeply from such real-world narratives, offering anonymised case studies that illuminate both exemplary and problematic disclosures. By dissecting these scenarios, showing the conversations that unfolded, revealing the letters exchanged, and offering practical tools shaped by lessons learned, the aim is to provide robust, accessible guidance that can empower clinicians and managers alike to act with confidence and compassion.

One such case involves a middle-aged patient undergoing elective surgery for what was expected to be a routine procedure. Shortly after the operation, an unexpected complication arose: a retained surgical instrument was inadvertently left inside the patient's abdomen. The surgical team quickly recognised the error during a follow-up imaging study and faced an immediate ethical and professional dilemma: how to disclose this serious mistake. The lead surgeon, in consultation with the hospital's duty of candour officer, immediately arranged a meeting with the patient and family members. The conversation was carefully planned, drawing on communication scripts developed through institutional training, emphasising honesty without overwhelming medical jargon, a sincere apology, and reassurance regarding the steps to rectify the problem. The disclosure was conducted face-to-face, creating space for questions, emotional responses, and shared decision-making about the next surgical intervention needed to remove the instrument. The patient's distress was met with empathetic listening and clear explanations outlining the safety checks that failed and how lessons would be applied to avoid recurrence. The documentation appended to the patient's records was meticulous, detailing the timeline, the disclosure conversation, and follow-up plans. This case illustrated how prompt, transparent communication combined with accountability and structured support can maintain trust even amid serious clinical error. It further underscored the importance of leaders fostering environments where staff feel secure, acknowledging mistakes without fear of disproportionate blame.

Contrast this with a case where the disclosure process faltered. A hospital encountered a medication error involving an overdose of a high-risk drug administered to an elderly patient. The adverse event resulted in prolonged hospitalisation and significant morbidity. Sadly, the initial disclosure was delayed; the healthcare professionals involved struggled with fear of litigation and reputational damage. When the disclosure finally occurred, it was performed via a hastily written letter lacking clarity and devoid of empathetic tone. The patient and family felt alienated, confused, and mistrustful. The lack of personal engagement and insufficient explanation compounded their distress, and the case attracted regulatory scrutiny. This example starkly illustrates how failing to meet the Duty of Candour standards promptly and compassionately can exacerbate harm not only physically but also psychologically and relationally. It highlights the vital need for structured protocols, staff training, and organisational cultures that support openness, ensuring disclosures are not seen as burdensome risks but as ethical imperatives that ultimately protect patients and providers alike.

Enriching these case studies are carefully constructed conversation scripts designed to guide clinicians through the delicate discourse of disclosure. These scripts balance candidness with sensitivity, encouraging professionals to prepare before speaking with patients. They recommend beginning with a clear explanation that an adverse event took place, expressing sincere regret, and providing detailed information about what is being done to address the situation. For example, a script might begin, "I want to talk to you about something important that happened during your care. We have found that an error occurred, and I am truly sorry for what you have experienced." Such phrases, though straightforward, require skilful delivery and emotional intelligence, as they set the tone for trust-building dialogue. The scripts also include guidance on responding to challenging emotions, anger, confusion, or grief, offering phrases like, "I understand this is distressing, and I am here to listen to your concerns and answer any questions." Importantly, the scripts stress the necessity to pause and allow patients space to process information, avoiding a rushed or defensive stance. These tools are invaluable for clinicians who may feel vulnerable or ill-equipped when faced with the daunting task of delivering difficult news, transforming a potentially fraught interaction into a healing moment.

Consent forms and templates for letters are integral components of effective disclosure practices and feature prominently in these case studies. Consent forms are designed not just as legal safeguards but as instruments to clarify patient understanding and agreement about further investigations or treatments following an adverse event. For instance, in one case, after disclosing an error that necessitated additional surgery, the clinical team provided a bespoke consent form that transparently detailed the risks, benefits, and alternatives to the corrective procedure. This ensured that the patient could make an informed decision grounded in full awareness, thereby respecting autonomy while fostering partnership. Letter templates, on the other hand, serve to communicate formally and compassionately when face -to-face meetings are unfeasible or as follow-up documentation after discussions. These letters carefully balance the need for transparency with appropriate reassurance, structured to include an apology, an account of what occurred, the remedial actions taken, and contact details for further dialogue or concerns. The letter's tone is designed to avoid defensive or legalistic language that might alienate recipients, instead canter the patient's experience and express genuine regret. When standardised and tailored thoughtfully, these resources streamline workflows and reinforce consistency in the organisation's approach to candour, mitigating variance that might otherwise confuse or distress patients and families.

Checklists emerge from these case analyses as practical instruments that break down the disclosure process into manageable steps, ensuring critical elements are not overlooked. For example, a disclosure checklist might begin with confirming the facts of the incident, notifying relevant team members and leadership, assessing patient risk and needs, scheduling disclosure meetings, preparing conversation points and documentation, and arranging immediate and longer-term support for all parties involved. Through one case study regarding delayed diagnosis, the implementation of a checklist dramatically improved the timeliness and quality of subsequent disclosures, ensuring that patients were engaged with empathy and clarity. The checklist also served as a protective framework for clinicians, signposting when to involve legal advice or management support, thus balancing transparency with procedural safeguards. Such structured approaches contribute toward normalising candour practices, embedding them into routine care rather than relegating them to crisis responses alone.

Critically, these anonymised case narratives reveal the nuanced emotional landscape that frames disclosures. Healthcare professionals frequently report fears of blame, shame, and legal repercussions, while patients and families often grapple with shock, betrayal, and grief. Successful disclosures acknowledge this emotional complexity, weaving compassion and honesty into every interaction. For example, a case depicting a nurse disclosing a medication mistake emphasised the value of vulnerability; the nurse candidly expressed personal sorrow alongside professional responsibility, which profoundly resonated with the patient's family and paved the way for reconciliation. Conversely, cases where disclosure felt mechanical or insincere tended to deepen wounds, undermining trust and sometimes prompting formal complaints. This emotional truth underscores that the duty of candour is more than a policy; it is a deeply human exchange demanding authenticity, courage, and kindness.

Further learning from these case studies touches upon the systemic changes catalysed by honest disclosures. In one situation, disclosure of a surgical site infection following a routine procedure led the hospital to institute a multidisciplinary quality improvement project targeting infection control protocols. Staff involved were encouraged to share insights without fear, fostering a culture where learning from harm was not only accepted but celebrated as a path to excellence. The leadership team used the event and its disclosure process as a touchstone for training across departments, linking the duty of candour with broader patient safety goals. This virtuous cycle of openness and improvement paints a compelling picture of how individual disclosures resonate far beyond immediate clinical encounters.

Finally, it is essential to recognise that these case studies are deeply contextual, influenced by the unique organisational culture, legal frameworks, and patient demographics within which they unfold. What works well in one healthcare setting may require adaptation elsewhere to resonate with local expectations and laws. Nevertheless, by critically analysing a range of situations from straightforward disclosures to complex ethical quandaries, this collection offers a foundational understanding and an adaptable toolkit. By internalising such lessons, healthcare professionals can approach their own duty of candour responsibilities not with trepidation but with a well-founded sense of preparedness and moral clarity, ultimately nurturing healthcare environments where transparency, trust, and patient-centred care flourish.

Conversation Scripts

In the delicate terrain of healthcare disclosure, the precise words spoken between clinician and patient can profoundly influence not only the emotional landscape of the encounter but also the trajectory of trust, healing, and resolution. The art of conversation in the moments following an adverse incident requires a rare combination of sincerity, clarity, empathy, and professionalism. As such, a repertoire of thoughtfully crafted conversation scripts serves as an invaluable resource to healthcare professionals navigating these difficult exchanges. These scripts present a range of scenarios from relatively straightforward disclosures to deeply complex conversations where emotions may run high and are designed to foster transparency and compassion while maintaining the integrity of clinical relationships. It is vital to recognise, however, that these scripts are not rigid templates but guiding frameworks, adaptable to the unique specifics of each case and the personalities involved. They embed core principles: acknowledgment of the event, an honest account without minimising or evading responsibility, attentive listening to patients' reactions and concerns, and a pathway toward support and follow-up.

For instance, consider the initial disclosure of harm to a patient when an unexpected complication arises during surgery, a scenario that demands careful balance between technical explanation and human connection. A conversation might begin by establishing a respectful and private setting, ensuring the patient feels safe to engage openly. "I want to talk with you about what happened during your operation today. There was an unexpected development that affected your recovery, and I believe it's important you understand exactly what occurred." This candid opening sets the tone for honesty while signalling the clinician's commitment to transparency. Following this, the clinician can proceed with a clear but non-technical explanation of the complication, pausing to gauge the patient's understanding and emotional response. The clinician might say, "During the procedure, there was a small injury to a nearby blood vessel, which means you might experience more bruising and a slightly longer recovery time. I understand this is upsetting news, and I want to make sure you have all the information you need." This passage models how medical jargon is tempered with accessible language and how space is intentionally given for the patient to absorb the information. Further, the clinician might then invite questions, showing openness to dialogue: "Please feel free to ask me anything, no matter how small or unclear it might seem. Your concerns are important to me."

In more challenging exchanges, such as when harm results from a preventable error or system failure, scripts emphasise not only acknowledgement of the event and its impact but also the clinician's ethical responsibility to apologise and discuss next steps. A powerful approach in such a setting might open with a statement of regret that is unambiguous yet compassionate: "I want to begin by sincerely apologising for what has happened. An error occurred, and I fully understand how this has affected you and your family." This is not a mere formality but a critical moment in rebuilding trust, where the clinician conveys accountability without defensive hedging. The conversation might then transition into explaining what is being done to address the issue and prevent recurrence: "We are conducting a thorough review to understand why this happened, and we are committed to learning from this so it doesn't happen again. Your safety is our highest priority." Alongside factual explanation, it is vital to recognise and validate the patient's feelings: "I can only imagine the frustration and disappointment you must be feeling. Please know that your experience matters deeply to us." This acknowledgement creates space for emotional expression, which can be further supported by attentive silence or gentle prompts if the patient is hesitant to speak. Clinicians can guide the discussion toward practical support by offering options for further medical care, counselling, or contact with patient liaison services: "We want to support you through this in any way we can. If you feel it would be helpful, we can arrange for you to speak with our patient advocate or a counsellor who specialises in helping families cope with difficult situations."

Another common yet sensitive context involves communicating unexpected deaths or irreversible harm. Here, the dialogue faces the dual challenge of delivering devastating news with as much gentleness as possible, while initiating the duty of candour process transparently but without overwhelming the patient or family members. A script for these moments carefully incorporates pauses, invites shared reflections, and avoids medical jargon that can alienate or confuse. The conversation might start with a compassionate disclosure: "I'm very sorry to have to tell you this, but despite our best efforts, [patient's name] has passed away." Following this, the clinician might express solidarity and sorrow: "I know how heartbreaking and difficult this is, and we want to be completely open with you about what happened." Once again, honesty remains paramount; the clinician can then outline the sequence of events in a clear, stepwise fashion, using phrases such as, "We want to explain to you exactly what we did and the challenges we faced to help you understand." Empathy is woven throughout as family members process shock or grief: "Please take your time – there's no rush to talk or ask questions now. When you're ready, we are here to answer anything you need to know." This flexible approach accommodates individual coping styles, whether immediate engagement or delayed discussion. Importantly, the script underscores offer of ongoing support, including bereavement services, counselling, and opportunities for follow-up meetings.

The practice of apology constitutes another cornerstone of duty of candour conversations, and scripts carefully reflect how to deliver an apology that is sincere, proportionate, and protective of professional boundaries. A template might gently remind the clinician to avoid language that admits legal liability prematurely, while still conveying empathy and responsibility: "I want to express my deepest apologies for what you have experienced. It was never our intention, and we are truly sorry that it happened. We are committed to understanding it fully and ensuring improvements." This delicate balancing act helps maintain the therapeutic alliance without compromising legal safeguards. The apology can be reinforced with an explanation of remedial actions underway and an invitation to collaborate with the patient or family on next steps: "We are taking this very seriously and are working with the whole team to make sure learnings are acted upon. If there is anything you would like us to know or support you with, please do tell us." Such wording affirms partnership and respect.

Equally instructive are scripts designed for disclosures in the presence of multiple family members, where dynamics are more complex, and emotions may clash. Here, the clinician's challenge includes managing diverse reactions while maintaining clear communication paths. A useful framework suggests beginning by acknowledging everyone's distress: "I can see this is a very difficult time for all of you, and I want to thank you for coming together to discuss this." Next, the clinician lays out the key facts as straightforwardly as possible, ensuring everyone hears the same version: "What happened was that [brief description]. You all must have the same information, so that I will explain it carefully." Throughout, the clinician observes for signs of misunderstanding or conflict, pausing to clarify or mediate if needed. To support emotional handling, scripts encourage phrases like, "I understand this news is hard to hear. Would anyone like to share how they are feeling or ask questions?" This invitation to voice emotions can facilitate mutual support among family members. When questions arise that require further detail or follow-up, clinicians can acknowledge the need for time and offer: "I want to make sure we find the right answers for you. Some information may require us to investigate further, and I will keep you updated every step of the way." This openness fosters confidence that nothing is being withheld.

Disclosures involving individuals with limited English proficiency or cultural differences introduce additional layers of complexity, prompting adapted scripts that emphasise clarity, respect, and cultural sensitivity. In these settings, the clinician recognises the essential role of trained interpreters rather than relying on family members to translate, ensuring accuracy and confidentiality. A conversation might commence with a warm greeting and assurance that professional interpretation is available: "We want to make sure you fully understand everything we are discussing today. An interpreter is here to help with any language needs." The clinician then proceeds slowly, avoiding idiomatic expressions and technical jargon, checking comprehension regularly by asking, "Does this make sense to you? Would you like me to explain anything again or differently?" Respectful acknowledgment of cultural values may follow: "We realise that in your culture, family decision-making is very important. Please let us know who we should involve when discussing next steps." Through these strategies, scripts promote inclusive, respectful disclosure that honours the patient's cultural context while fulfilling candour responsibilities.

One of the most recurrent challenges depicted in conversation scripts entails managing patients or families who express anger, blame, or distress at the disclosure. In these emotionally charged moments, clinicians must maintain composure, validate feelings without defensiveness, and avoid escalation. Scripts often recommend phrases such as, "I can see how upsetting this is for you, and your feelings are completely understandable. I want to listen and support you through this." If anger surfaces sharply, the clinician might gently suggest a pause or a short break: “I want to make sure we have the best possible conversation, so if you'd like, we can pause for a moment and continue when you're ready.” Such pauses provide emotional space and can prevent conversations from deteriorating. Maintaining a respectful and calm tone while reiterating the commitment to transparency and safety reassures patients and families that their concerns are being taken seriously. When accusations or demands for immediate answers arise, scripts guide clinicians to acknowledge limits realistically: “We want to give you full answers, and some things take time to investigate properly. I promise we will keep you informed as we learn more.” This honesty, paired with regular updates, reduces uncertainty and frustration.

Beyond initial disclosures, conversation scripts also address conversations around consent for further investigations, tests, or participation in root cause analyses. These scripts balance the need for patient autonomy with a clear explanation of the potential benefits and risks of further steps. A clinician might begin, “To understand fully what happened, we would like your permission to review your medical records and speak with everyone involved in your care. This helps us learn and improve safety.” Such a request is framed to emphasise partnership and collaboration. The clinician anticipates and responds to common questions or concerns: “You might wonder if this will affect your care or privacy. Please be assured that all information is handled confidentially, and your care will continue uninterrupted.” Tailoring the conversation to reassure and inform fosters trust and participation.

Moreover, the scripts encourage healthcare professionals to provide closure while leaving the door open for ongoing dialogue. After the key points of disclosure, apology, and support options have been conveyed, a closing might sound like: “Before we finish, is there anything else you would like to talk about or ask? It’s important to us that you feel heard and understood. If you think of questions later, please don’t hesitate to reach out to the team or me.” This invitation acknowledges the often-evolving process of adjustment and ensures patients and families do not feel abandoned once the immediate disclosure conversation concludes.

Embedded within these conversation scripts are subtle but essential cues for clinicians to observe their own language, tone, and body language, as well as the physical environment where disclosures occur. Scripts reinforce the value of quiet, private spaces free from interruptions, unhurried time frames, and the clinician’s presence being fully attentive and undistracted. Even the pauses, the timing of silences, and gentle eye contact form an unspoken language that supports the verbal content. For example, a scripted phrase followed by a deliberate pause allows the patient the moment to absorb difficult information rather than feeling rushed or overwhelmed. Scripts may include gentle prompts to normalise patients’ feelings: “It’s perfectly natural to feel upset or confused right now.” These empathetic insertions help humanise what can otherwise be clinical or intimidating conversations.

The integration of these scripts into clinical practice often involves rehearsing scenarios, role-playing with colleagues, or using them as reflection tools after actual disclosures. By practising these conversations, healthcare professionals build confidence and familiarity, equipping themselves to respond sensitively and effectively under pressure. The scripts also highlight the iterative nature of dialogue; it is rarely a one-off event but part of an ongoing process of communication, reassurance, and shared decision-making. This longitudinal approach recognises that healing and restoration of trust take time, and each conversation, scripted or improvised, contributes to the broader journey.

Incorporated within the book's practical tools, these conversation scripts are presented alongside checklists that prompt clinicians to prepare for disclosure discussions thoroughly, identifying key points to cover, anticipating questions, and ensuring support systems are in place. Sample phrases are accompanied by contextual notes encouraging adaptation to individual circumstances, such as age, cognitive capacity, or existing relationships. Where appropriate, scripts demonstrate the staged nature of disclosure from the initial conversation to follow-up meetings to updates on investigation outcomes, thus framing candour as a continuum rather than a single event.

Taken together, the conversation scripts form a vital bridge between abstract principles of openness and the gritty reality of human interaction in times of vulnerability and uncertainty. They affirm that while no single script can guarantee a perfect conversation, approaching disclosures with sincerity, preparation, and empathy dramatically enhances the likelihood of a meaningful and healing encounter. With thoughtful language and genuine care, healthcare professionals can transform the trauma of harm into a shared moment of respect and commitment to improvement, ultimately reinforcing the integrity and humanity at the heart of medicine.

Templates and Checklists

In the complex and often emotionally charged environment of healthcare, the availability of structured, ready-to-use practical tools can be invaluable for professionals navigating the Duty of Candour. Transitioning transparency into action demands more than just goodwill; it requires meticulous preparation and clear frameworks to ensure that disclosures are managed consistently, compassionately, and compliantly. In this section, we provide an array of refined templates and carefully designed checklists that serve as navigational aids through the multifaceted processes of incident reporting, patient communication, and organisational compliance. Each instrument is crafted to empower healthcare professionals with clarity and confidence, balancing the needs of the patient, the integrity of the healthcare system, and the unique professional obligations incumbent upon clinicians and managers alike.

One of the foundational tools offered is a range of conversation scripts crafted with psychological insight and communication theory to help clinicians approach difficult conversations with patients and families. These scripts are not rigid formulas but rather adaptable frameworks designed for flexibility based on the context. They emphasise empathetic listening, transparent disclosure of facts, sincere apologies, and collaborative planning for remediation and future prevention. For example, an initial disclosure script begins by setting a tone of genuine empathy, recognises the patient's distress, and clearly but sensitively outlines what is known about the incident and what is still under investigation. It encourages validating the emotions of patients and families before progressively guiding the dialogue toward acknowledgment of harm and assurance of commitment to safety improvements. Such scripts integrate subtle language choices proven to reduce defensiveness and help maintain trust, enabling candour without sacrificing professional composure or increasing exposure to legal risk.

Complementing these verbal scripts are templates for formal written communications, including letters of disclosure, apology letters, and notifications of incident investigations. These documents are structured to maintain clarity and precision while avoiding unnecessary jargon that can alienate or confuse recipients. For instance, the apology letter template guides the author in expressing accountability without admitting legal liability in explicit terms, combining warmth with prudent language. This balance ensures that patients feel heard and respected, which is foundational for healing and reconciliation. Another template organises the notification letter to regulators and key stakeholders, ensuring compliance with legal timeframes and fulfilling the ethical responsibilities required under most healthcare systems. By adhering to these templates, healthcare professionals can avoid common pitfalls such as vague language or overlooked details that might otherwise complicate subsequent investigations or legal proceedings.

Alongside communication aids, this compendium includes consent forms tailored to the disclosure process itself. Recognising that transparency sometimes prompts patients or their families to request involvement in investigations or to seek further information under privacy laws, these forms assure a clear understanding of what participation entails. They establish patient expectations about confidentiality, the scope of shared information, and the limits of disclosure within regulatory constraints. The use of such consent structures mitigates misunderstandings and fosters a partnership model that respects patient autonomy without overwhelming clinical staff or legal teams with ambiguous obligations. By incorporating consent forms that explain the process in layperson language and provide space for patient queries, healthcare providers create a safer foundation for meaningful dialogue beyond the initial disclosure.

Checklists form the backbone of these tools, supplying a sequential roadmap for both immediate responses and longer-term follow-up actions after an adverse event. These checklists mitigate the risk of human error or oversight by ensuring that every critical step from initial fact-gathering, patient notification, multidisciplinary team meetings, documentation, to final reporting is accounted for. They serve multiple audiences, with distinct versions tailored for frontline clinicians, management teams, and risk or legal departments. For example, a clinician's checklist reminds the professional to confirm the patient's identity, document the incident thoroughly in real time, conduct the disclosure meeting as soon as feasible, and arrange for support services such as counselling. Meanwhile, managerial checklists focus on policy adherence, resource allocation for investigations, and preparation of internal and external reports. These tools foster accountability and help embed the Duty of Candour into the organisational culture, transforming abstract responsibility into concrete action.

One particularly useful checklist included guides healthcare teams through the emotional and logistical complexities of delivering a face-to-face disclosure meeting, helping staff anticipate and prepare for a range of patient reactions, including anger, grief, or confusion. It prompts clinicians to review not only the factual timeline but also pertinent non-verbal communication strategies, ensuring body language conveys openness and sincerity. It encourages planning for multidisciplinary attendance where necessary, such as involving a senior clinician, nurse, and patient advocate or chaplain. This approach reassures patients and families that their concerns are respected and taken seriously by the entire care team. The checklist also reminds healthcare professionals to document the meeting meticulously afterward, recording both the dialogue and emotional dynamics, which can be critical for ongoing care and organisational learning.

Another critical tool presented is a detailed reporting checklist designed to ensure comprehensive submission to regulators and legal authorities in jurisdictions with mandatory reporting requirements. This checklist breaks down the elements needed for transparency, from patient identifiers and incident timelines to corrective actions and preventive measures instituted. It also features troubleshooting tips for handling incomplete information or conflicting accounts, guiding teams to maintain integrity without speculation. By embedding legal compliance within everyday workflows, this checklist reduces the burden on overstretched staff and minimises the risks of regulatory penalties or reputational damage. Through its systematic approach, it encourages continuous reflection on safety improvements grounded in open disclosure.

To facilitate organisational learning, a checklist devoted to investigative processes helps guide multidisciplinary reviewers through compiling evidence, conducting interviews, and analysing root causes. It prompts teams to remain objective and avoid assigning blame prematurely, focusing instead on systems improvements. The tool encourages setting clear timelines for investigation milestones and defining responsibilities to prevent delay. It integrates recommendations for involving patient representatives in a way that respects confidentiality but enhances transparency. This balance is crucial for turning adverse events into constructive learning opportunities. Moreover, the investigative checklist supports documentation that is incident-specific but also generalised enough to feed into broader risk management databases, fostering a culture of continuous improvement.

Augmenting these procedural instruments, templates for policy development and review provide healthcare leaders with foundations for creating or updating their organisational approaches to Duty of Candour. These template policies balance regulatory demands with practical implementation strategies and incorporate examples of best practices drawn from diverse healthcare settings. The inclusion of model statements on leadership commitment, training requirements, and staff support mechanisms encourages the establishment of open environments where candour is normalised rather than feared. Furthermore, guidance is embedded within these templates to adapt for varying cultural or system-specific nuances without diluting core principles of transparency, integrity, and patient-centredness. Leaders can thus build or refine frameworks knowing they conform to evolving legal landscapes while meeting frontline realities.

All these tools are designed to be customisable, recognising the diversity of healthcare environments and emergent needs. They are provided in formats conducive to electronic health record integration or easy printing, ensuring accessibility during high-pressure moments. Practical tips accompany the tools, such as reminders to keep copies securely but accessibly stored, suggestions for training staff on their use, and advice on periodic review to reflect changing regulations or organisational lessons learned. As such, these templates and checklists are not static but living documents meant to evolve alongside the institution's culture and external requirements.

Finally, within the broader narrative of practising Duty of Candour, these practical tools emphasise that candour is not an afterthought nor an administrative hurdle but an ethical and professional imperative that must be seamlessly woven into everyday clinical practice. When used effectively, they transform daunting conversations and complex processes into manageable, human-centred interactions framed by respect and transparency. This can greatly ease the anxiety healthcare workers face around disclosures, reduce the potential for conflict or litigation, and most importantly, support patients and families through some of their most vulnerable moments with honesty and care.

By integrating these templates and checklists into healthcare practice, individuals and organisations affirm their commitment to openness, safety, and continuous improvement. They herald a system where, when things do go wrong, responses are swift, compassionate, and transparent. This collection equips healthcare professionals not only to meet the letter of legal duties but to embody the spirit of candour that sacred trust between provider and patient is vital for healing to occur beyond physical treatment. In this way, Duty of Candour evolves from policy into culture, and from obligation into opportunity.

Appendices: Checklists, Sample Letters, Policy Templates, Further Reading

Disclosure Checklists

In the delicate and often emotionally charged landscape of healthcare, the process of disclosure after an adverse event is a critical juncture that demands clarity, compassion, and precision. To navigate this complex terrain with confidence and integrity, healthcare professionals benefit immensely from having reliable, detailed checklists that outline each essential step of the disclosure process. These checklists serve not only as practical guides but also as reassuring companions, reminders of obligations and best practices that reinforce a culture of transparency and respect. The disclosure checklist begins long before the conversation with the patient or family actually takes place; it starts with the internal acknowledgement and swift recognition of the incident that has occurred. This initial step involves alerting the relevant clinical and managerial teams, ensuring patient safety is immediately prioritised, and gathering reliable information about what transpired. It also demands a rapid assessment of the clinical and legal implications of the event, as well as identifying the appropriate spokesperson or team who will lead the disclosure. Before any communication happens, the healthcare professional must be thoroughly briefed and oriented to key facts, potential risks, and the patient's current condition. This preparation ensures that disclosure is grounded in honesty but also calibrated to provide clarity without overstepping uncertain boundaries.

Once the groundwork has been laid, the checklist moves toward planning the disclosure conversation itself, emphasising the creation of a supportive environment where the patient or family feels safe and respected. Deciding on a suitable setting, ideally private, quiet, and devoid of interruptions, is a crucial detail often overlooked in the rush to communicate. The timing of the disclosure, too, must balance urgency with sensitivity; while honesty must not be delayed, rushing can undermine the patient's ability to process information and respond. The checklist invites professionals to consider who else should be present: should other clinical team members attend to provide technical information? Would a patient advocate or support worker be helpful? Prepping the patient by informing them in advance that a discussion about their care is due has been shown to soften sudden shock and open pathways for dialogue rooted in trust. These preparatory steps cultivate a foundation of psychological safety, enabling the disclosure to unfold with genuine empathy rather than a defensive posture.

At the heart of the checklist is a detailed guide for the disclosure conversation itself, a stage imbued with ethical weight and emotional intensity. The checklist underlines the necessity of beginning with clear, straightforward language that avoids medical jargon, carefully situating the event within the patient's care timeline and explaining what occurred without minimising or exaggerating. It stresses the importance of using "I" statements rather than depersonalised phrasing, which empowers healthcare professionals to take ownership and humanise the dialogue. Throughout this exchange, active listening is paramount; the checklist advises pausing frequently to allow patients and family members to respond, acknowledging their feelings, questions, and concerns with sincere validation. It also encourages transparency about what remains unknown, avoiding the temptation to offer premature conclusions or speculative details that could later complicate trust. The checklist recognises that disclosure conversations are rarely linear and advises flexibility in managing moments of silence, distress, or anger with calmness and reassurance, and steering the dialogue back to key points with gentle prompts if confusion arises.

Integral to the disclosure process outlined in the checklist is the provision of a thorough apology. Far from being a mere formality, the apology serves as an authentic expression of regret and a bridge toward healing. The checklist details how to deliver this apology with appropriate language that takes responsibility without admitting legal liability, which is a subtle but vital distinction. It underscores timing, suggesting that the apology should not be perfunctory but delivered at a moment when the recipient can genuinely absorb it. The professional is also guided to address what steps will be taken in response, including immediate remedial actions and longer-term plans to prevent recurrence. Offering information about support services such as counselling, patient advocacy, or second opinions is positioned as an essential element of compassionate disclosure, recognising that patients often need resources to cope with the aftermath beyond the factual explanation.

Following the disclosure conversation, the checklist insists on meticulous documentation, which is foundational for accountability and learning. Every aspect of the conversation, from the initial recognition of the adverse event to the specifics of what was communicated, must be recorded comprehensively and contemporaneously. This documentation is not a mere bureaucratic exercise; it forms a legal record and a valuable tool for reflection and quality improvement. The checklist provides detailed prompts for this documentation: noting the date, time, participants present, content shared, patient responses, emotional dynamics, and any follow-up arrangements. It also reminds clinicians to use objective language and avoid judgments or subjective assessments that could be misconstrued. If the disclosure conversation results in any changes to the patient's care plan or referral to specialist services, these updates must be clearly documented and communicated to all relevant healthcare providers to uphold continuity and safety.

Another critical element woven through the disclosure checklist is engagement with regulators and legal counsel when appropriate. While openness remains the central value, there may be cases requiring nuanced interaction with legal teams to balance candour and risk management. The checklist guides when to escalate incidents for regulatory review and how to ensure compliance with statutory duty of candour requirements specific to different jurisdictions. It advocates for timely and transparent reporting to external bodies while safeguarding patient confidentiality and minimising unnecessary distress. For healthcare leaders, this portion of the checklist becomes a vital strategic tool, enabling them to monitor organisational adherence and foster systemic improvements based on incident data.

The checklist also thoroughly addresses the follow-up phase, acknowledging that disclosure is not a single event but an evolving process. Patients and families often require ongoing communication, as new information becomes available or as they seek clarification and restitution. The checklist encourages scheduling review meetings, providing written summaries as needed, and offering clear channels for feedback and questions. It highlights the importance of continuous emotional support, both for those affected by the event and for the healthcare staff involved, whose well-being is crucial for sustaining a culture of candour. Recognition of the psychological impact on clinicians, sometimes referred to as secondary trauma or moral injury, is woven into the checklist to ensure a holistic approach to healing and learning.

Throughout all these stages, the disclosure checklist is permeated by a spirit of cultural humility and adaptability. The checklist reminds practitioners to consider the patient's cultural background, health literacy, and personal preferences in how disclosure is conducted, advocating for flexible communication styles and the use of interpreters or cultural liaisons when necessary. It discourages a one-size-fits-all approach, inviting professionals to tailor their methods with sensitivity and respect for diversity, which enhances trust and mitigates harm.

Embedded within the disclosure checklist is also a focus on learning and system improvement that transcends individual events. Each incident and its disclosure process becomes a pivotal case study for refining policies, training, and practices. The checklist advises recording lessons learned, convening multidisciplinary review meetings, and revising protocols as needed. Its stepwise layout ensures that disclosure is not an isolated ethical act but an integral component of institutional quality and safety systems. In fostering this mindset, the checklist contributes to shifting healthcare culture from blame to one of shared responsibility and continuous improvement.

The practical force of these checklists is further amplified when paired with corresponding conversation scripts, template letters, and sample policies. Together, these resources help healthcare professionals prepare thoroughly and navigate even the most difficult interactions with increased confidence and empathy. They help demystify the complex emotional and procedural choreography of disclosure, transforming it from a daunting obligation into an achievable practice rooted in human connection and professional integrity.

In summary, the disclosure checklists compiled in this book serve as indispensable roadmaps for clinicians and healthcare leaders alike, clarifying each essential step from recognising an adverse event through to concluding follow-up and systemic learning. By harmonising ethical principles, legal obligations, communication skills, and organisational requirements into a coherent and accessible framework, these checklists empower professionals to perform the duty of candour with clarity, compassion, and courage. They embody the very spirit of transparency that is foundational to patient-centred care, reinforcing that when things go wrong, honest and thoughtful disclosure is not only a professional responsibility but also a profound opportunity to rebuild trust, foster healing, and cultivate safer healthcare environments for all.

Sample Letters and Forms

In the delicate landscape of communicating adverse events, the importance of well-crafted, thoughtful written correspondence cannot be overstated. Sample letters and forms serve as vital tools enabling healthcare professionals to navigate the complex emotional and legal terrain with confidence and clarity. These templates act as blueprints carefully designed to balance transparency, empathy, professionalism, and compliance. They provide structure in the midst of vulnerability, ensuring that every word contributes meaningfully to fostering trust and alleviating patient and family distress. While the content of each letter or form must be personalised to the specific incident and relationship, having a reliable foundation guides healthcare professionals in honouring their Duty of Candour responsibly and compassionately.

Among the most essential of these communications are initial notification letters, which represent the first step of disclosure to patients or their families after an adverse event occurs. These letters are critical because they set the tone for future interactions; they must be clear, direct, yet deeply respectful. Constructed carefully, they acknowledge the incident promptly without overwhelming recipients with medical jargon or unnecessary detail. They begin by identifying the purpose of the letter to inform the recipient that an event affecting their care has taken place and establish a commitment to openness by affirming that the healthcare team is dedicated to providing ongoing information and support. By framing the disclosure in an empathetic tone and outlining next steps, these letters serve as a bridge from uncertainty to dialogue, ensuring patients feel seen and valued rather than sidelined.

Following initial notifications, apology letters are another cornerstone of effective communication in duty of candour practices. An apology in healthcare is more than a mere formality; it is a profound expression of empathy that acknowledges harm and the resulting emotional impact. A well-articulated apology letter conveys genuine regret without admitting fault prematurely or exposing the practitioner to undue legal risk. Templates in this category provide carefully balanced wording that respects both ethical imperatives and practical considerations. They avoid defensiveness and defensive language while reaffirming the commitment to investigate the event thoroughly and to learn from it. These letters also frequently invite dialogue, encouraging patients and families to share their concerns or ask questions, thus fostering a collaborative spirit rather than an adversarial one. The use of simple, heartfelt language helps reduce feelings of alienation and demonstrates that the healthcare provider honours the patient's experience and dignity.

Beyond direct patient communication, internal forms and checklists play a vital role in systematising the duty of candour process. These documents ensure that disclosures comply with institutional policies as well as legal and regulatory obligations. For instance, incident reporting forms, designed specifically to capture relevant details of what occurred, who was involved, and what immediate actions were taken, serve both as documentation and as tools for quality improvement. Templates for these forms include fields that prompt thoroughness without being burdensome, providing a consistent framework for healthcare professionals to record facts, human factors, and contextual elements objectively and promptly. The structure supports transparency internally by fostering accountability and helping managers monitor compliance with disclosure timelines and support interventions.

In addition to incident reports, action plan templates are invaluable in demonstrating a healthcare organisation's commitment to learning from adverse events. These forms guide teams through root cause analysis documentation, enabling systematic identification of not only what went wrong but why. Within the context of duty of candour, sharing these findings with the patient and family, when appropriate, epitomises transparency and stewardship. Action plan documents typically include sections for describing corrective measures, assigning responsibilities, and setting deadlines, facilitating tangible improvements that enhance patient safety. When patients see that an incident has spurred meaningful reflection and change, it nurtures their trust and reassurance that their suffering has led to positive transformation.

Policies and procedural templates included in the appendix support healthcare managers and leaders in embedding the duty of candour into organisational culture. These policy documents outline the ethical rationale, legal requirements, and operational protocols for disclosures, providing healthcare staff with clear expectations and guidance. The templates may include definitions of terms related to duty of candour, steps required for reporting and disclosure, responsibilities of various roles, and categories of incidents that mandate disclosure. They also address nuances such as handling concerns over legal liability, documentation standards, and escalation pathways. Importantly, these templates emphasise compassionate communication as foundational, encouraging organisations to blend compliance with humanity. By offering a consistent, accessible resource, these policies help foster a normalised environment where candour is not feared but embraced as a core element of patient-cantered care.

The practical utility of conversation scripts cannot be overstated and is therefore emphasised within the suite of templates. While the book already discusses communication skills in detail, these scripts serve as hands-on tools for healthcare providers preparing for difficult discussions. They scaffold the conversation with suggested phrasing for introductions, setting agendas, acknowledging emotions, and responding to questions or concerns. These scripts are crafted to accommodate common scenarios, including initial disclosures, delivering apologies, discussing investigation outcomes, and arranging follow-up meetings. They serve both as rehearsal aids and real-time guides, helping clinicians maintain composure, clarity, and empathy even when emotions run high. Scripts subtly remind professionals to validate feelings, avoid blame, and remain honest about uncertainties, all while reinforcing respect and partnership with the patient or family. The provision of multiple scripted variations allows for adaptation to different contexts and cultural sensitivities, supporting personalised yet principled communication.

In preparing and sharing these written materials, attention to tone is paramount. The templates consciously avoid language that might feel cold, legalistic, or bureaucratic. Instead, they adopt a warm, sincere, and respectful voice that prioritises the human experience of harm. They acknowledge the vulnerability patients and families endure when confronting unexpected adverse events and communicate an unwavering commitment to listening and improving. Simultaneously, wording is carefully chosen to maintain professional boundaries, ensuring that apologies and explanations do not unintentionally admit liability in a way that jeopardises healthcare providers' legal positions. The balance is subtle but essential and thus reflected in multiple drafts of each template to accommodate different jurisdictional requirements and institutional cultures.

Particular attention is paid to the sequencing and timing articulated within the templates. For example, initial notification letters and scripts emphasise delivering information as soon as practically possible after the incident is recognised, with assurances that further information will be provided as investigations proceed. Apology letters frequently follow once facts have been verified, allowing for appropriate expressions of regret grounded in an accurate understanding of the event, while still ensuring empathy is evident from the outset. Checklists remind healthcare teams to complete each step within prescribed time frames, reinforcing promptness without sacrificing thoroughness. This structured timing helps mitigate anxiety for all involved and signals respect for the patient's or family's need to know without delay.

In addition to templates for individual communication, the appendices guide documenting conversations and disclosures. Documentation forms include prompts for noting not only what was said but how it was received, any questions asked, and plans for follow-up. This detailed recording supports continuity of communication across providers and departments as well as compliance with regulatory oversight. It also protects clinicians by evidencing that candour was exercised diligently and respectfully. In settings where multiple healthcare professionals engage with the patient or family, unified documentation preserves clarity and minimises contradictory messaging.

Furthermore, certain templates focus on consent and confidentiality considerations inherent in disclosure communications. These forms guide practitioners in explaining patients' rights regarding personal health information, including the extent to which incident details can be shared with family members or other parties. They assist in navigating sensitive boundaries while upholding transparency, thus respecting autonomy and privacy simultaneously. Incorporating such elements into disclosure protocols prevents misunderstandings and fosters trust that sensitive information is handled with integrity and care.

The appendices also feature letters tailored to particular contexts, such as communication with regulators or legal advisors. These templates facilitate timely, accurate reporting and collaboration, ensuring that duty of candour obligations extend beyond the immediate patient-provider relationship to encompass broader accountability. They provide language to acknowledge regulatory requirements without compromising patient confidentiality or the sanctity of investigative processes. By harmonising internal disclosures with external communications, healthcare organisations maintain credibility, avoid sanctions, and promote system-wide patient safety enhancements.

To support ongoing professional reflection and development, the appendices include curated further reading lists and resource links. These encompass relevant legislation, ethical guidelines, case law summaries, and communication training materials. Encouraging healthcare professionals to update their knowledge and skills continually complements the practical assistance offered by the templates. Access to rich reference material fosters a learning mindset vital to sustaining a culture of candour and compassion over time.

In summary, the collection of sample letters and forms acts as a comprehensive toolkit empowering clinicians, managers, and leaders to practise the Duty of Candour with dignity, clarity, and confidence. By providing carefully designed, adaptable templates for every step of disclosure from initial notification, through apology, investigation reporting, and policy implementation, this resource transforms the abstract ideal of candour into a pragmatic reality. These materials enable healthcare professionals to communicate transparently and empathetically even in the most challenging circumstances, build and maintain patient trust, and contribute meaningfully to organisational learning and patient safety. Ultimately, incorporating these templates into everyday practice is an essential pillar supporting the overarching goal of fostering healthcare environments where openness and honesty are not just obligations but shared values.

Policy Templates and Further Reading

In any comprehensive guide to practising the Duty of Candour, supporting documents and resources hold a critical place, acting both as practical tools and as foundational pillars that reinforce confidence, clarity, and consistency. These materials, meticulously crafted and thoughtfully curated, serve to bridge the often-intimidating divide between theoretical principles and actionable daily practice. To begin, detailed checklists for disclosure steps provide a roadmap that ensures no essential element is overlooked when an adverse event occurs. These checklists are designed to be intuitive yet exhaustive, encapsulating everything from the initial recognition of the incident to the final stages of follow-up and documentation. By using these stepwise guides, healthcare professionals can better manage the immediate emotional and procedural challenges that arise, securing a structured approach to transparency that simultaneously respects the timeline and sensitivities involved. The power of such checklists lies not merely in their ability to remind or organise but in their role as a stabilising force; clinicians and managers can lean on these frameworks during moments of stress, reducing the risk of errors or omissions in communication that might otherwise compound harm to patients and families.

Flowing naturally from the procedural checklists, sample apology letters form an essential resource that embodies not only candour but also the human connection that must permeate such disclosures. Crafted with care and sensitivity, these templates illustrate how to balance honesty with empathy, transparency with compassion, and professionalism with warmth. They offer a starting point, not a rigid script from which healthcare providers can personalise their communication to fit each unique context and relationship. The letters avoid jargon and legalese, encouraging straightforward language that respects the intelligence and emotional state of recipients. They emphasise acknowledgment of harm, expression of regret, and reassurance of commitment to learn and improve. Importantly, these templates also model appropriate tone and boundary-setting, aiming to prevent defensiveness or blame-shifting while fostering trust and hope. For healthcare workers unfamiliar or uneasy with apologising, having such letters on hand demystifies the process and provides an empowering sense of preparedness, enabling them to initiate difficult conversations with greater ease and integrity.

Policy templates tailored to healthcare settings constitute another indispensable component of this resource repository. These are crafted to assist organisational leaders and managers in embedding duty of candour standards into their institutional fabric, ensuring that the principles are not just personal responsibilities but collective commitments. These policies cover a spectrum of essential domains, including the criteria for disclosure, responsibilities at various hierarchical levels, timelines for action, coordination with legal and regulatory bodies, and mechanisms for staff support. The templates provide clear language yet remain adaptable, acknowledging the diversity of healthcare contexts from small community clinics to large academic hospitals and the varied legal frameworks governing different regions. In addition to articulating procedural mandates, these documents underscore the cultural and ethical ethos that should animate every disclosure process: valuing openness, fostering safety, and promoting learning. By adopting and customising such policies, healthcare organisations manifest their dedication to transparency not only in words but through resolute structural support, setting a tone that pervades daily operations and encourages continuous improvement.

Beyond procedural and policy aids, the appended further reading sections open doors to a richer, multi-dimensional understanding of the Duty of Candour. These thoughtfully compiled bibliographies and resource lists invite readers to delve deeper into foundational theories, emerging research, and multidisciplinary perspectives that enrich comprehension and practice. They include seminal texts on medical ethics, landmark legal cases shaping disclosure norms, psychological insights into communication after harm, and leadership studies focused on cultivating open cultures. Journals, articles, and podcasts featured provide ongoing updates and diverse viewpoints, reflecting the evolving nature of both healthcare practice and societal expectations. By guiding readers toward these resources, the book fosters intellectual curiosity and lifelong learning, recognising that effective candour is a dynamic skill honed over time through reflection and engagement with new ideas. Practitioners are thereby encouraged not to see disclosure as a static checkbox but as an evolving dialogue shaped by scholarship, experience, and humane innovation.

When these documents coexist as a comprehensive suite of thoughtfully interlinked checklists, apology letter templates, organisational policies, and reading materials, they form a cohesive ecosystem that supports not only immediate action but also sustained cultural change. They enable healthcare professionals to navigate the complexities of adverse events with pragmatic confidence and emotional intelligence, integrating legal, ethical, and interpersonal dimensions seamlessly. More than just appendices, these resources embody the spirit of the Duty of Candour, transforming abstract commitments into living practice. In doing so, they help to dismantle barriers of fear and mistrust, fostering environments where openness is not a risk but a strength, and where the painful realities of harm become opportunities for genuine connection and healing.

It is important to highlight that these templates and checklists are designed with adaptability in mind. Healthcare environments vary enormously in terms of size, specialty, patient demographics, and available resources, so one size does not fit all. The policy templates encourage organisations to engage their diverse stakeholders, clinicians, managers, patients, and legal advisors in iterative refinement processes, ensuring documents reflect local values, norms, and legal requirements. This collaborative tailoring strengthens buy-in and accountability, making policies living documents rather than static mandates. Similarly, sample apology letters, while standardised to foster best practices, are best utilised as guides rather than scripts, inviting personalisation that respects individual communication styles and the idiosyncrasies of each incident. The further reading recommendations are curated to incorporate a global perspective, acknowledging differences in cultural understandings of candour and varying healthcare system structures, thus expanding the scope of learning beyond any one jurisdiction.

The checklists, in particular, deserve elaboration regarding their functional breadth. They span phases from initial incident identification, urgent safety measures, immediate and transparent communication with patients and families, documentation requirements, involvement of organisational and external oversight, provision of support to staff affected by the incident, and mechanisms for identifying systemic improvements. Each step includes guidance on timing, content focus, and responsible parties, designed to ensure clarity and precision in execution. The emotional and ethical challenges implicit in disclosure are also addressed, with prompts reminding practitioners to assess patient and family readiness to receive information, to use compassionate language, and to document discussions comprehensively without compromising privacy or legal concerns. The checklists also nurture interprofessional collaboration by defining clear roles for clinical frontline workers, risk managers, and senior leadership, promoting synchronised efforts that span the entire incident response continuum.

Sample apology letters incorporated within the appendices demonstrate balanced candour, offering an acknowledgment that is honest about what is known and unknown, accepting responsibility where appropriate without self-incrimination, expressing genuine empathy, and highlighting the commitment to learning and preventing recurrence. The letters advise tactful phrasing to navigate complex dynamics, such as when patient harm is multifactorial or when investigations are ongoing.

They include examples of both initial apologies made verbally and formal written communications that may follow. Acknowledging the legal sensitivities around admissions of fault, these templates foreground transparency and humanity without undermining necessary professional caution. Sample letters also accommodate various scenarios, ranging from minor incidents with no lasting harm to serious events requiring multidisciplinary disclosure meetings, offering adaptability for different clinical realities.

Policy templates included serve as foundational frameworks from which institutions can build or enhance their own duty of candour protocols. These documents carefully integrate national and regional legal mandates with ethical standards recommended by professional bodies to ensure comprehensive compliance. They delineate escalation procedures, ensuring clarity on when and how incidents must be reported internally, how regulators are involved, and under which circumstances legal counsel should be sought. Furthermore, the policies emphasise mechanisms for supporting staff well-being during disclosure processes, recognising the emotional toll on caregivers and outline training requirements that ensure all employees understand their roles in upholding candour. Attention is given to embedding feedback loops that enable learning from incidents to be documented, shared, and acted upon systematically, moving beyond isolated events towards organisational resilience. The templates also underscore the importance of leadership commitment in shaping organisational culture, mandating regular audits of compliance and quality improvement metrics related to transparency initiatives.

The further reading resources compiled in the appendices forge an intellectual scaffold that underpins the practical tools. They include classical works on medical ethics, such as seminal essays on the principles of beneficence, non-maleficence, and autonomy, which form the ethical backdrop against which the Duty of Candour is understood. Legal commentaries provide insight into evolving jurisprudence about disclosure and liability, helping practitioners navigate the often-delicate balance between openness and risk management. Communication research featured highlights techniques for managing difficult conversations, delivering bad news, and negotiating misunderstandings with emotional intelligence and cultural sensitivity. Leadership literature explores how to transform organisational cultures to value psychological safety and transparency, essential ingredients for meaningful candour beyond mere compliance. Furthermore, case studies from diverse healthcare systems offer comparative perspectives on what has worked, what challenges remain, and how innovation continues to drive better practices worldwide. Curated journal articles and guidelines from authoritative bodies provide updated evidence-based recommendations, reinforcing the evolving nature of this important field.

The incorporation of digital resources and online platforms among further reading selections recognises modern learners' preferences and needs. Webinars, podcasts, and interactive learning modules are referenced to facilitate flexible, engaging education on the duty of candour. These multimedia formats often include role play, scenario-based learning, and reflective exercises that complement the more traditional written texts. They are invaluable for reinforcing theoretical knowledge and fostering the practical skills necessary to approach disclosure with both competence and compassion. Healthcare teams are encouraged to use these resources not just individually but as parts of group training sessions, fostering shared understanding and collective commitment that translate into the everyday culture of the organisation.

Ultimately, the appendices and supporting documents are not mere add-ons but integral to fostering a sustained and embedded culture of candour. They move the abstract ideals of transparency and trust from aspiration into actionable reality, furnishing healthcare professionals with tangible, user-friendly tools that anticipate the complexities and demands of real-world clinical environments. By facilitating timely and honest communication, encouraging personalised yet principled apologies, guiding institutional policy formation, and widening access to ongoing learning, these resources are a beacon of clarity and reassurance amid the uncertainty following adverse events. They acknowledge the profound human impact of these moments not only on patients and families but on caregivers and organisations offering pathways toward healing, learning, and improvement.

As a final thought, the availability of these documents encourages a proactive rather than reactive approach to candour. Institutions and individuals are urged to familiarise themselves with these resources well before difficult incidents arise, integrating them into training programs, simulations, and continuous professional development. This preparedness nurtures resilience and empowers healthcare professionals to face challenging conversations with a steadiness rooted in knowledge, empathy, and integrity. Moreover, it signals a commitment to patients and their families that openness and accountability are not isolated acts but enduring values woven into the very fabric of care. The act of making these resources accessible, visible, and routinely used creates an environment where candour is normalised, reducing fear and stigma, and ultimately advancing safer, more humane healthcare systems for all.

www.ingramcontent.com/pod-product-compliance
Lightning Source LLC
LaVergne TN
LVHW060042210926
848481LV00013B/3936